COGNITIVE THERAPY OF SCHIZOPHRENIA

Guides to Individualized Evidence-Based Treatment

Jacqueline B. Persons, *Series Editors*

Providing evidence-based roadmaps for managing real-world cases, volumes in this series help the clinician develop treatment plans using interventions of proven effectiveness. With an emphasis on systematic yet flexible case formulation, these hands-on guides provide powerful alternatives to one-size-fits-all approaches. Each book addresses a particular disorder or presents cutting-edge intervention strategies that can be used across a range of clinical problems.

Cognitive Therapy for Schizophrenia
David G. Kingdon and Douglas Turkington

Treating Bipolar Disorder: A Clinician's Guide to Interpersonal and Social Rhythm Therapy
Ellen Frank

Cognitive Therapy of Schizophrenia

David G. Kingdon
Douglas Turkington

Series Editor's Note by Jacqueline B. Persons

THE GUILFORD PRESS
New York   London

Library of Congress Cataloging-in-Publication Data

Kingdon, David G.
    Cognitive therapy of schizophrenia / David Kingdon, Douglas
Turkington.
        p. ; cm. — (Guides to Individualized Evidence-Based Treatment)
    Includes bibliographical references and index.
    ISBN 1-59385-104-9 (alk. paper)
    1. Schizophrenia—Treatment.   2. Cognitive therapy.
    [DNLM: 1. Schizophrenia—therapy.   2. Cognitive Therapy—methods.
WM 203 K52c 2005]   I. Turkington, Douglas. II. Title. III. Series.
    RC514.K5653 2005
    616.89′806—dc22
                                                                2004012738

About the Authors

David G. Kingdon, MD, is a psychiatrist working with a mental health team in the U.K. National Health Service and is a Professor at the University of Southampton, United Kingdom. He has published many papers, chapters, and books about cognitive therapy of severe mental illness and mental health service development over the past several decades. Dr. Kingdon has also been involved in developing policy for mental health services as an advisor with the Department of Health in the United Kingdom and as chair of the Council of Europe's Expert Working Group on Psychiatry and Human Rights.

Douglas Turkington, MD, is a liaison psychiatrist working at the Royal Victoria Infirmary in Newcastle-upon-Tyne, United Kingdom. He is also Senior Lecturer at the School of Neurology, Neuroscience and Psychiatry of the University of Newcastle-upon-Tyne. Dr. Turkington is a founding fellow of the Academy of Cognitive Therapy and has lectured and given workshops on the subject of cognitive-behavioral therapy (CBT) for schizophrenia for the last 15 years. He continues to collaborate with cognitive therapists from the Newcastle Cognitive Therapy Centre to develop and test new CBT approaches to psychotic symptoms. He has also project-managed a major pragmatic trial of the delivery of CBT by psychiatric nurses to schizophrenic patients in the community. Dr. Turkington's other major research interests include schema vulnerability and psychotic symptom content, working with posttraumatic stress disorder and social anxiety in schizophrenia, and the development of techniques to improve adherence and negative symptoms.

113058

Series Editor's Note

Many mental health practitioners view schizophrenia as unresponsive to any therapy save medication. In fact, this is not the case. People who have schizophrenia benefit from several psychosocial treatments, including social skills training, token economy programs, interventions to reduce expressed emotion in the patient's living setting, and psychoeducation (Kopelowicz, Liberman, & Zarate, 2002). This book presents one of the newest evidence-based psychosocial interventions for schizophrenia: cognitive therapy. Cognitive therapy, like the other psychosocial interventions, allows patient and therapist to roll up their sleeves and really grapple with debilitating symptoms that are too often seen as incomprehensible and untreatable from a psychosocial perspective.

This book is the inaugural volume of the series titled "Guides to Individualized Evidence-Based Treatment." The books in this series aim to facilitate the transportation of evidence-based therapies from the ivory tower to the front lines of clinical settings. Toward that end, this volume, like the others in this series, describes in some detail not just the interventions of the therapy, but also the conceptualizations upon which the interventions are based. With this information, clinicians will not blindly carry out interventions, but will be guided by a conceptualization they can use to adapt the treatment to the needs of the patient at hand in a way that is flexible yet systematic and theory driven (Persons, in press). Kingdon and Turkington present clear cognitive-behavioral conceptualizations of schizophrenia at the level of the disorder, the subtype, and the symptoms (e.g., hallucinations).

This volume provides invaluable assistance to the clinician who works with schizophrenic patients. In addition, as a clinician who works with (nonschizophrenic) anxious and depressed patients, I found this book unexpectedly illuminating. Ideas presented here for conceptualizing and managing negative symptoms of schizophrenia have been useful in my work with depressed patients who do not respond to other evidence-based interventions, and with personality-disordered individuals who struggle with paralyzing passivity. Ideas presented here have also been helpful in treating the psychotic symptoms experienced by patients with borderline personality disorder and bipolar disorder, and in treating patients with anxiety disorders, body dysmorphic disorder, eating disorders, and depression, who frequently display thinking that is delusional or nearly so. In the past, whenever I encountered psychotic symptoms in my patients, my first thought was "medication needed." I tended to throw up my hands and refer the patient out to a psychiatrist. After reading this book, my responses to psychotic symptoms are quite different. Although, of course, medications remain an important intervention option, now when I encounter a psychotic symptom, my first thought is, "How can I conceptualize this symptom using cognitive-behavioral models, and what interventions does that conceptualization suggest?" Wow. For this reason, I found the symptom-level formulations and interventions presented here to be particularly fascinating and useful.

This volume is authored by two gifted clinicians whose writing conveys their deep understanding of schizophrenia and their respect for those who suffer from it. The authors also communicate their commitment to helping these individuals manage their symptoms in order to live a meaningful and gratifying life. Some individuals with schizophrenia can accomplish these goals without medication; in general, however, the evidence indicates that at the current point of our knowledge, most patients with schizophrenia need medication in addition to psychosocial treatment in order to function at their best.

It is my pleasure to congratulate David Kingdon and Douglas Turkington on a fine book that will make an important contribution to the treatment of patients suffering from schizophrenia and schizophrenic symptoms.

JACQUELINE B. PERSONS, PhD
San Francisco Bay Area Center
for Cognitive Therapy

REFERENCES

Kopelowicz, A., Liberman, R. P., & Zarate, R. (2002). Psychosocial treatments for schizophrenia. In P. E. Norman & J. M. Gorman (Eds.), *A guide to treatments that work* (2nd ed.). New York: Oxford University Press.

Persons, J. B. (in press). Empiricism, mechanism, and the practice of cognitive-behavior therapy. *Behavior Therapy*.

Preface

This manual is a guide to cognitive therapy with people who have schizophrenia. We describe an approach that is consistent with current research evidence of the effectiveness of cognitive therapy in schizophrenia and stresses the role of a collaboratively generated formulation in guiding the process of therapy. It may also be useful in the management of psychotic symptoms complicating the management of other conditions, such as depression, social phobia, obsessive–compulsive disorder, posttraumatic stress disorder, and borderline personality disorder, but the evidence of effectiveness in these areas is less. The psychotic symptoms of schizophrenia have traditionally been viewed as biological phenomena linked to an underlying but as yet unknown disease process. As a consequence, traditional teaching programs have included statements that these symptoms are not psychologically understandable and are unresponsive to any kind of psychological intervention. This is equivalent to suggesting that the only possible approach to, for example, a "stroke" (cerebrovascular accident) is drug treatment, whereas it is well accepted that developing ways of coping and building up strengths through physiotherapy can lead to considerable gains. Cognitive therapy may help in a similar or even more fundamental way in schizophrenia, supplementing any beneficial effects of medication.

However, many practitioners continue to believe that the content of psychotic symptoms should be ignored and that any psychological work or engagement attempted with psychotic symptoms is liable to lead to increased distress and exacerbation of symptoms, as a result of having opened up disturbing areas. This perspective has meant that people with schizophrenia have had few opportunities to explore and understand these distressing and debilitating symptoms. They have also not been encouraged to use their own internal resources to manage their distressing symptoms and even test out the validity of their beliefs because it has not been believed that this could help. Physicians thus have had no alternative but to progressively increase antipsychotic medication. This might have some additional effects but often simply leads to further distress from side effects, especially akathisia (so-called restless legs), and disability through other side effects (sedation, tremor, weight gain, impaired concentration and memory).

Yet over the past decade, much has changed about the way we understand schizophrenia and how we can make a major difference in the distress and disability it causes. Chapter 1 provides information focused on the disorder and the ways in which cognitive therapy has improved our understanding of schizophrenia, its associated symptoms, and the clinical subgroups of which it consists. Its relationship to other mental health problems, such as depression, anxiety, phobias, and borderline personality disorder, is also explained. Since the early 1990s, behavioral and later cognitive techniques have been found to be effective in reducing distress and the burden of symptoms. Positive and negative symptoms, depression, and insight have been shown to improve through the use of cognitive and behavioral techniques, and this effect has also proved to be durable over the short term. (Chapter 2 describes the evidence for this.) This led to the development of cognitive models explaining the form, content, onset, and maintenance of symptoms. Such cognitive models have drawn on vulnerability–stress conceptualizations and contributions from the cognitive models of depression, intrusive thoughts, panic, and trauma, including consideration of vulnerability from the underlying beliefs that shape attitudes toward relationships.

Cognitive therapists assess collaboratively with the person who has schizophrenia, and often the person's caregivers, his or her specific needs and experiences (Chapter 5) and then develop individually generated formulations (described in Chapter 6). Symptoms, in this case psychotic ones, become increasingly comprehensible, both in form and in content. The prescriptive—or "cookbook"—approach to therapy has been replaced by the targeted use of techniques that are formulation-congruent—that is, jointly developed by the client and therapist and appropriate to the quality of the therapeutic relationship (the theme of Chapter 4). Involving and orienting the client to different ways of approaching personal difficulties needs careful consideration that is dependent on the care setting and the resources available (Chapter 7). The use of formulation-based cognitive therapy in schizophrenia has led to its becoming an ideal adjunct to low-dose antipsychotic medication, psychoeducation (especially with normalization; Chapter 8), and work with caregivers. Techniques for dealing with delusions (Chapter 9), hallucinations (Chapter 10), and other thought disorders (Chapter 11) are now available. Negative symptoms are no longer an area of therapeutic nihilism, as strategies with a growing evidence base are available to work with them (Chapter 12), and also with comorbid conditions such as depression and substance misuse (Chapter 13). Cognitive therapy can play an important role in early intervention efforts (Chapter 3), and issues relating to relapse prevention and termination of therapy are discussed as well (Chapter 14). Should difficulties happen to persist or depart from the usual pattern of treatment, some supplementary approaches are also described (Chapter 15).

Psychological nihilism in psychosis is now being replaced by therapeutic optimism. People with schizophrenia and psychotic symptoms and their caregivers can now reasonably expect mental health services to deliver a balanced, integrated, effective, and understandable service. We hope this manual will help you to do so.

Acknowledgments

We would like to thank Jacqueline B. Persons, Series Editor, and Kathryn Moore, Executive Editor of The Guilford Press, for inviting us to contribute and for their invaluable assistance in shaping the book and commenting on succeeding drafts. Many people have contributed to the development of cognitive-behavioral therapy for people with schizophrenia and are named in the References and Further Readings, but Aaron Beck's support, influence, and encouragement need to be particularly acknowledged. Most important, thanks are due to all the patients who have taught us so much over the years about their often very distressing but sometimes uplifting experiences and their ways of understanding and living with them.

Contents

COGNITIVE THERAPY OF SCHIZOPHRENIA

ONE

What Is Schizophrenia?

Schizophrenia has been problematic in terms of causation and classification since it was first described over a century ago, initially as dementia praecox. It has also become a very stigmatized and misunderstood condition. Schizophrenia can now be diagnosed reliably using criteria developed over the past few decades and is recognized as a diagnostic entity by international classification systems. However, the diagnosis covers a very diverse group of individuals who present in a variety of ways and require a wide range of therapeutic approaches—indeed, Bleuler (1911), when he first used the term, referred to it as "the group of schizophrenias." As a result of the diversity of presenting symptoms, Persons (1986) and Bentall and colleagues (1988) have argued the case for focusing on individual symptoms such as hallucinations, delusions, and thought disorder rather than on diagnosis. There is also an intermediate position that considers possible clinical subgroups within the overarching schizophrenia diagnosis (described in detail later in this chapter). Schizophrenia can therefore be viewed from three vantage points: disorder, subtype, and symptom.

These approaches can be considered complementary:

- The broad diagnostic category "schizophrenia" has been useful for communication, education, and research purposes. Information about research into characteristics of people with schizophrenia (e.g., age of onset) and their outcomes with treatment is given in this and the next chapter.
- Subgroups provide a way of unifying symptom clusters to further guide therapy where the condition is so diverse in presentation. For example, hallucinations can occur in different circumstances and be linked to different symptoms. They may be abusive and very distressing and require direct work on the effects of trauma. Alternatively, they can support a systematized set of paranoid delusions (e.g., voices attributed to "the CIA"), and the primary focus will then be on dealing with the beliefs underlying the delusional system rather than much direct work on the voices.
- A focus on individual symptoms is also valuable. Identifying symptoms is relatively straightforward. Therapy focused on symptoms is simple to understand and can be used in psychological management based on an individualized case formulation.

1

This chapter describes:

1. The characteristics of schizophrenia, including symptoms and demographic information
2. The cognitive model of schizophrenia, which draws on vulnerability–stress conceptualizations of schizophrenia involving the interaction between
   • Biological, social, and psychological vulnerabilities and
   • Individual stresses or stressful circumstances
3. Clinical subgroups of schizophrenia with illustrative cases
4. Ways of understanding psychotic symptoms

CHARACTERISTICS OF SCHIZOPHRENIA

The course of schizophrenia is reasonably well understood but unfortunately has changed little over time. New treatments, both pharmacological and psychosocial, may be beginning to have an impact on this, but it is too early to be demonstrable. Of those who develop the illness, traditional teaching has been that approximately 20% make a full recovery, 20% have relapses with no intervening deterioration, 40% have relapses with some deterioration, and fewer than 20% remain chronically ill and show little recovery. There is some evidence (presented below) that this may be a gloomier picture than the reality. However, there is no question that the clinical presentation of schizophrenia to clinicians is a variable one that hinges strongly on the stage of the disorder and the mixture of symptoms.

Symptomatology

People with schizophrenia tend to experience a variety of psychiatric symptoms, including certain types of hallucinations (particularly auditory, visual, and somatic—i.e., causing physical sensations), delusions, thought disorder, and loss of insight. These symptoms usually coexist with negative symptoms (alogia, affective blunting, poor motivation, and social withdrawal; see the definitions and explanations later and in Chapter 12), which can be either primary or secondary to depression or medication side effects. Cognitive deficits—interference with thinking—such as disturbed attention, impaired short-term memory, and poor recognition of facial expressions also occur and lead to or perpetuate poor coping abilities and social isolation.

Schizophrenia has been defined by the presence or absence of specific symptoms. A combination of these symptoms and a measure of duration is necessary to make the diagnosis, according to criteria established by the *International Classification of Diseases* (10th edition; ICD-10; World Health Organization [WHO], 1992) and the American Psychiatric Association's *Diagnostic and Statistical Manual of Mental Disorders* (4th ed., text rev.; American Psychiatric Association [APA], 2000). ICD-10 requires one very clear-cut schizophrenic symptom or two less clear symptoms to have been present most of the time for a duration of 1 month. DSM-IV-TR requires one characteristic symptom to have been present for a significant proportion of time for a 1-month period or two less characteristic ones (see APA, 2000, for further details).

Symptoms used for diagnostic purposes include:

- Hearing his or her own thoughts spoken aloud.
- Third-person hallucinations (voices talking about him or her).
- Hallucinations in the form of a running commentary on what he or she is doing or thinking.
- Somatic hallucinations (experiencing feelings that are believed by the person to originate externally but to others do not appear to do so).
- Delusions of thought withdrawal or insertion (beliefs that others can remove thoughts from, or put them into, a person's mind).
- Delusions of thought broadcasting (the belief that his or her thoughts are broadcast to others).
- Delusional perception (when the person sees or hears the same thing as other people but attaches a meaning to it that is delusional, i.e., not shared by others).
- Delusions of passivity ("made" acts, thoughts, or emotions—when the person is convinced that he or she is being made to do, think, or feel things by an external force or by other people when this does not appear to be the case).

Negative symptoms and the medium-term course of the disorder are included in the diagnostic criteria of DSM-IV-TR but not ICD-10. The introduction of such classificatory systems has improved reliability, but the validity of the diagnosis remains in question. In other words, it is now possible to get good agreement on whether someone has signs and symptoms that characterize schizophrenia, but there is still uncertainty about how meaningful a diagnosis (or group of diagnoses) it is in terms of putative causes, prognosis, or treatment response. Prior to the advent of stricter criteria during the 1970s, schizophrenia was diagnosed much more often in the United States as compared to Europe. With the introduction of agreed-upon criteria and major international studies, it has become clear that the incidence of schizophrenia is much the same throughout the world, although there are a small number of groups who do have higher rates (Boydell et al., 2001).

Many other symptoms occur as well as those that are used in diagnosis, and these may be as distressing and disabling, or even more. These include psychotic symptoms such as abusive or command hallucinations (in the second person—e.g., "You're useless" or "Kill yourself") and thought disorder—where the train of thought is very difficult to follow—and nonpsychotic symptoms such as depression, anxiety, obsessions, compulsions, social phobia, and agoraphobia.

Demographics

Of the general population, 0.5–1% will develop schizophrenia at some point in their lives, although the rate of onset of schizophrenia is quite low (10–20 cases per 100,000 population per year). There is no difference in rates between men and women, but women have a mean age of onset 3–4 years later than their male counterparts. The rate of incidence is higher in urban than in rural areas. Social outcome in developed countries, as opposed to that in less developed countries, has generally been conceived as poor, with episodic relapse or chronic deterioration and heightened suicide risk. People with schizophrenia have a higher-than-expected mortality rate, owing to a number of different causes, with suicide accounting for some of the difference. Young men with relapsing schizophrenia and evidence of repeated self-harm are particularly at risk.

Schizophrenia is arguably the most debilitating psychiatric disorder—psychologically, financially, and socially. It is the 13th most expensive illness in terms of health expenditures, according to the World Bank. The traditional view has been that people suffering from this disorder are seldom employed, are unlikely to develop meaningful relationships, and have a tendency to drift down through the social classes into living in isolation or even on the streets. But this negative view has been repeatedly challenged. A study of people who had been diagnosed as having schizophrenia recently showed that approximately 50% of them, at 15-year and 25-year follow-up, had favorable clinical outcomes (Harrison et al., 2001). Whatever the long-term perspective, much of the workload of community mental health teams involves working with people with schizophrenia and related diagnostic categories (schizoaffective disorder, bipolar disorder, and delusional disorder).

THE COGNITIVE MODEL OF SCHIZOPHRENIA

Models used to explain schizophrenia have been based on biological, social, and psychological conceptualizations (see Table 1.1). Biological models have emphasized physical causes for the disorder, including abnormalities in structure and function caused by, for example, genetics, birth injury, abnormal development, or viral influences. Social models have focused on environmental influences, including poverty, influences of the inner city and culture, and family and societal pressures. Psychological models have taken a variety of perspectives, often considering complexities in interpersonal relationships.

None of these models has found universal acceptance since all of them have limitations in explaining the available research findings or in being substantiated by them. As a result, models incorporating elements of each have been proposed—based on the interactions between vulnerabilities and stress. These vulnerabilities may have a biological origin (e.g., genetic predispositions), may be inborn psychological characteristics, or may result from social circumstances during intrauterine or early development. Stresses also can be biological (e.g., infection or drug intoxication), psychological, or social. Cognitive models of delusions have recently been set forth by Garety and col-

---

TABLE 1.1. **Vulnerability–Stress Model of Psychosis**

Psychotic symptoms, including those of schizophrenia, arise from a combination of *vulnerabilities*:

- Biological, including genetic
- Social, including living in an urban environment
- Psychological, which may include:
  —An externalizing bias
  —A tendency to "jump to conclusions"
  —Difficulty in "taking the role of the other"
  —Negative or confusing underlying beliefs about the self

with *stress* that is *significant to the individual* because of its type, severity, associations, or possible implications and that may be amplified by a fear of "madness" and stigmatization.

---

leagues (2001) and Beck and Rector (2002), and of hallucinations by Morrison (1998). These syntheses are based on a biopsychosocial model and attempt to include and explain recent research findings.

Biological Vulnerabilities

Schizophrenia certainly has a genetic component in terms of vulnerability. This may be due to a small number of genes acting independently on a "multiple-hit" basis with an additive effect. Evidence of a genetic contribution, or predisposition, to schizophrenia derives from studies of identical and nonidentical (monozygotic and dizygotic) twins. The risk of developing schizophrenia is nearly 50% among children both of whose parents have schizophrenia. One influential follow-up study of twins found that both developed schizophrenia in 36% of the cases where the twins were identical, while for nonidentical twins the figure was 14%. This confirms the importance of heritability in schizophrenia, but since only just over a third of those who are genetically identical develop the disease there must also be an important environmental component to etiology. Confirmation of a genetic proclivity also derives from adoption studies, where it has been demonstrated that twins bought up in different environments have similar (i.e., higher-than-normal) rates of schizophrenia to those bought up together. There are some problems with these studies, in part attributable to other linked factors—for example, a tendency for mothers with schizophrenia to receive poorer antenatal care and a lack of reliability in diagnoses in studies. Twins are also clearly unusual in many ways, and their identity issues in particular may affect their susceptibility to schizophrenia. Viewed from the other direction, 89% of people with schizophrenia will have parents who do not have schizophrenia, 81% will have no affected first-degree relative, and 63% will show no family history of any kind of the disorder. So, the current consensus is that there is a genetic vulnerability in some people with schizophrenia that is probably due to multiple genes acting independently, with an additional environmental component.

Schizophrenia also carries a biological predisposition linked to birth trauma and maternal viral infection. Geddes and Lawrie (1995) estimated that complications in pregnancy and delivery may increase the incidence of schizophrenia by 20%. More specifically, Verdoux and colleagues (1997) found that subjects with onset of schizophrenia before age 22 were three times more likely than those with onset at a later age to have had a history of abnormal presentation at birth and 10 times more likely to have had a history of complicated cesarean birth. The risk of developing schizophrenia for people with obstetric complications, such as prolonged labor (which can cause oxygen deprivation), is four times greater than those who have none, and a history of such complications has been found in 40% of those with schizophrenia. A complicating factor here is that those with schizophrenia have an increased likelihood of obstetric complications due to psychosocial factors.

There is also a seasonal effect: People who develop schizophrenia are more likely to have been born in the late winter or spring. Epidemics of viral illnesses such as measles, influenza, and chickenpox have been shown to correlate with an increase in the numbers of births of people who later develop schizophrenia. The increased risk of developing the illness in this way is probably very small. However, these risk factors may combine with genetic risk to create significant vulnerability to schizophrenia. Individuals with schizotypal personality traits (eccentric behavior with anomalies of thinking and affect) are overrepresented in the families of people with schizophrenia, possibly showing that these personality traits may be markers of an underlying vulnerability or independent risk factors. Findings of brain changes in groups of people with schizophrenia, such as increased ventricular size, may also manifest themselves through increasing vulnerability.

Yet many individuals with schizophrenia appear to have no obvious biological or genetic predisposition. In such cases, personal, social, or psychological vulnerability linked to early life traumas or disturbance may be linked to the development of schizophrenia in later life.

Social Vulnerabilities

Schizophrenia is commoner in cities than in rural areas, and this seems to hold true even when a tendency for people who become ill to move from the country into cities is taken into account. Other vulnerabilities, as mentioned previously, are most likely to develop in inner-city areas where there is limited access to or use of obstetric facilities. Such areas also tend to have high levels of deprivation and abuse of various types, leading to increased stress and possibly the formation of negative schemas (e.g., related to paranoia), which tend to perpetuate psychotic symptoms. These are also the very areas where there is easier access to hallucinogenic drugs, which can likewise activate and perpetuate symptoms. Finally, inner-city areas are often inhabited by new immigrant peoples and asylum seekers, who have a higher incidence of schizophrenia. This particularly occurs in second-generation immigrants, possibly because of their struggles in relation to cultural conflicts, alienation, racism, and limited support.

Psychological Vulnerabilities

Certain psychological vulnerabilities that may predispose individuals to schizophrenia have been described over the past decade. Processes leading to cognitive distortion may be present, such as tendencies to externalize praise for good events or blame for negative events, and to personalize that praise or blame to one individual or group (Bentall & Kinderman, 1998). Externalization and personalization are linked to "theory of mind" deficits. Basically, these deficits involve a pervasive problem in empathy (i.e., an inability to take the role of other people and understand their perspectives). They may also be "self-serving," in that paranoid thinking may be defensive or functional (effective) in reducing discrepancies between the "actual self" and the "idealized self." Persons with schizophrenia may protect self-esteem by making external causal attributions for negative events (Bentall & Kinderman, 1998)—that is, blaming others for things that go wrong, rather than themselves. Some people with schizophrenia may have a propensity to develop delusions or hallucinations as a way of protecting against unbearable affect or loss of self-esteem (Turkington & Siddle, 1998), rather than, for example, becoming anxious or depressed. Delusions may be marked by systematization and often grandiosity, which protect the persons against underlying beliefs such as "I am worthless," "I am damaged," "I am unlovable," and "I am evil."

Comparisons have been drawn between intrusive thoughts in panic and obsessive–compulsive disorders on the one hand, and psychotic symptoms on the other (Morrison, 1998). In both instances, intrusive thoughts are unwanted or unacceptable to the persons experiencing them and are perceived as uncontrollable. The essential difference between hallucinations and obsessions is that the former are attributed externally (i.e., are seen as coming from outside the mind), while the latter are attributed internally (Kingdon & Turkington, 1998). Morrison (2001) argues that positive symptoms can be conceptualized as intrusions into awareness, and that a vulnerability to misinterpretation of these causes the associated distress and disability.

People with certain paranoid delusions display typical cognitive distortions. These typical distortions include making arbitrary inferences (drawing conclusions from inadequate information) and holding those conclusions more firmly than others would (Garety & Freeman, 1999). Such delusions are formed as attempts by people who are suffering from symptoms (e.g., voices or physical symptoms of anxiety) to make sense of them in an absence of knowledge about them. They are typically culturally syntonic (e.g., alien abduction, satellite control, torment with lasers).

Chadwick and colleagues (1996) have also described a tendency for different groups of clients to view themselves or others negatively—as illustrated by the terms "poor me" or "bad me." These psychological characteristics may be genetically determined vulnerabilities, but it is also possible that they are the results of specific stressors or circumstances in earlier life or a combination of these. It is certainly the case that the circumstances in which persons find themselves, and the prevailing cultural beliefs, both influence the content of the persons' own beliefs and the degree of conviction with which these are held.

Stressors

Stressful life events and circumstances can take a variety of forms. These can be obviously distressing (e.g., bereavements and other losses) or less so (e.g., changing from the day shift to the night shift, or moving away to college). They can include the effects of hallucinogenic drugs and alcohol as independent and contributory stressors. Some people may be particularly sensitive to these stresses at certain times during their lives or because of life circumstances or previous significant events.

People with critical and abusive auditory hallucinations with linked depression and low self-esteem often disclose during therapy that they have been the victim of childhood sexual abuse or adolescent trauma, including bullying. Early trauma has been linked to hallucinations in schizophrenia (Heins, Gray, & Tennant, 1990) and specifically to diagnostic symptoms of schizophrenia (Ross et al., 1994). In such cases it may be a further negative life event that triggers abusive voices. Such hallucinations may also exist for many years before the person presents for services, but eventually they become intolerable or the person makes a decision that the time has come—sometimes even because he or she is only now strong enough—to deal with them. These voices are often the voice of the abuser or, for example, people who have strongly criticized or bullied the client, and often there are linked visual hallucinations or imagery.

There is often strong avoidance of inquiry and disclosure and avoidance of working with the traumatic material by both the client and the clinician. The increased arousal of the traumatized state worsens the hallucinatory experience, as does any linked sleep deprivation. Both of the above can lead to the emergence of obsessional thoughts often with linked compulsive rituals. In such cases a systematic guided formulation linked with the abuse-congruence of the psychotic symptom content will often allow the person to begin the process of reevaluating the trauma and of working with the linked distress through the beliefs involved—for example, shame, anger, and unworthiness. People with such distressing symptoms may have repeated readmissions, suicidal attempts, and high suicide risk due to the combination of critical and command hallucinations and linked depression. Trauma can also follow the experience of psychosis through additional personal victimization. Many of our vulnerable clients are targets for muggings, beatings, and sexual assaults and repeated abusive relationships (Walsh et al., 2003). Again, these are often not elicited or disclosed but act to exacerbate hallucinations, persecutory delusions, and negative symptoms.

Perhaps the most powerful maintaining factor is the person's belief about the psychotic symptoms amplifying any distress intrinsic in the stressful experience itself. People who believe that their voices are omniscient or omnipotent, as is often the case (Birchwood & Chadwick, 1997), tend to activate particularly poor coping strategies. This includes especially those who believe that the voice is that of a powerful spiritual being such as God or Satan. On the other hand, Romme and Escher (1989) showed that optimal coping was linked to much less threatening explanations, for example, "repressed voices from my childhood," "part of my personal development," "a parapsychological gift . . . like a medium." Biological explanations are helpful to some people who feel less ashamed and more in control when they have an "internal/medical" explanation. Many people, however, feel disempowered, alienated, and depressed by holding this belief. The crucial thing is to work with the client's beliefs about symptoms if they are dysfunctional and, if need be, to work toward a new belief that best suits the individual.

Vulnerability–Stress Model

The vulnerability–stress hypothesis of schizophrenia simply states that vulnerabilities and stresses combine to produce the symptoms characteristic of the disorder. The precise symptoms (e.g., voices or delusions) and combination of symptoms (e.g., any of the clinical subgroups described later) that are produced will be determined by the nature of the vulnerabilities and stresses experienced. People with vulnerabilities from genetic weighting, poor obstetric care, and negative schemas may become psychotic through the occurrence of environmental stressors such as drug use, trauma, or the accumulation of social problems. The negative schemas, lack of support, use of hallucinogens, and generally impoverished social environment with victimization then act to maintain psychotic symptoms.

In addition to such background factors, fear of the experience of psychotic symptoms can exacerbate stress. The experience of transient psychotic symptoms such as paranoid ideas and auditory hallucinations is surprisingly common in apparently healthy community samples (Johns & Van Os, 2001). Such "psychotic" symptoms are as common as obsessional thoughts and are usually interpreted in a similarly negative manner. This is particularly so in Western culture, where such symptoms are perceived in a highly stigmatized way. A person who develops pseudohallucinations due to sleep disturbance linked to pressure of work could interpret the transient symptoms as follows:

> "I'm sure I heard someone speak just now . . . They seemed to be calling my name . . . Am I starting to go nuts? . . . If I have a breakdown, I will lose my job . . . What will people think of me? . . . Maybe I will be put in a mental hospital . . . I will be locked up and injected . . . Life will be unbearable."

This sequence of increasingly anxious interpretations of the original experience can lead to increased anxiety and further sleep deprivation. This process can act to maintain and exacerbate the hallucinatory experience. The person can begin to become convinced that he or she is fundamentally different from others—"schizophrenic," "mad"—and this can then be reinforced by others' responses. Normalizing (see Chapter 8) provides information about circumstances where such experiences occur—for example, to people under extreme stress, such as hostages—and is understandable as related to those stressful experiences. The people experiencing such circumstances are different in terms of the distress they are undergoing but not fundamentally different "as people." The message is that given sufficient or specific types of stress, most individuals—maybe everyone—could develop the symptoms the person is experiencing.

There is therefore a clear rationale for the use of normalizing explanations (Kingdon & Turkington, 1994) as an early strategy in engagement and therapy with the psychotic person. Normalizing leads to reduced anxiety and improved collaboration. It can also lead to an early success experience due to reduction in hallucinatory intensity by reducing the anxiety that can be acting as a maintaining variable. Other psychotic symptoms (e.g., thought insertion and ideas of reference) are often the subject of similar catastrophization and can be helped through normalizing explanations.

Instead of (or as well as) catastrophizing about psychotic and panic symptoms, people can also become actively involved in pursuing "safety behaviors" in each of these disorders, especially with voices (Morrison, 1998). These are designed by the person to reduce the impact of the symptoms he or she is experiencing, but as these behaviors tend to use avoidance primarily, they can instead lead to their increase or at least persistence. The symptom is interpreted in these circumstances as a danger signal. The person will not engage with or take ownership of the experience and will avoid any situation where the voice might occur. If hearing the voice tends to occur in social situations, then the person will strenuously avoid social contact. When safety behaviors are deployed in this way, the hallucinations never have the opportunity to be extinguished and are actively maintained by the coping style of the person. When there is exacerbation of the experience of the psychotic symptoms by catastrophization and the use of safety behaviors, intense and disabling psychotic experiences can develop. The safety behaviors are only stopped when more functional coping strategies have been collaboratively developed and have shown efficacy in symptom management when used in graded homework exercises or during the session itself. Normalizing explanations and the use of voice diaries that encourage engagement and the gradual dropping of safety behaviors can then be effectively used together.

Change may therefore occur through the client's understanding the way in which his or her vulnerabilities and the stresses he or she has experienced interact. This sense of understanding has two effects:

1. It draws meaning from confusion, which is reassuring and destigmatizing: "I'm not that different from everyone else," "now I understand why I feel so bad."
2. It provides the basis for specific interventions that can alleviate the distressing and disabling symptoms, for example, problem solving, coping with voices, and testing out strong beliefs and working with their consequences.

CLINICAL SUBGROUPS

Crow (1985) described positive and negative syndromes (Type 1 and Type 2) of schizophrenia and suggested that different neurological mechanisms might underlie the two syndromes. Prominent negative symptomatology at the time of the first episode that does not resolve during the index admission has been shown to predict a poor outcome (Carpenter et al., 1988). Barnes and Liddle (1990) posited a three-factor model of chronic schizophrenia involving perceptual distortion (i.e., the presence of delusions and hallucinations), disorganization (i.e., thought disorder), and negativity. Bleuler (1911) initially described a "group of schizophrenias," and sporadically since that time subgroups have been delineated, such as simple, paranoid, hebephrenic, and catatonic schizophrenias, but such distinctions have had little impact on clinical practice.

Cognitive therapy involves careful investigation of initial episodes, and it has become apparent to us over the past few years that there are at least four common presentations that seem to require similar individual management plans, though with distinctions from one group to another (Kingdon & Turkington, 1998, 2002). Validation of these groups has been through review of clinical cases and discussion at many workshops and lectures; participants have generally agreed that the descriptions of these groups are clinically recognizable and fit with aspects of people with schizophrenia with whom they have worked. More formal research into the groups is currently being pursued. They are described here, with case examples, and used throughout this manual to help clarify the management of a complex heterogeneous group of people.

Sensitivity Psychosis

People with sensitivity psychosis—who tend to present as adolescents or young adults—experience gradual onset, usually over a period of a year or more, in which they seem to have increased difficulty in managing events that they find to be stressful, for example, social situations, academic study, leaving home, or breakdowns in relationships (see Table 1.2). Sometimes they have been quite successful at school, although perhaps a bit solitary, or they may in contrast have had serious problems coping previously but remained in normal education or low-grade work. There have, however, been changes that they have experienced as stressful, for example, changes in jobs or in their educational setting.

Psychotic ideas emerge, sometimes transiently, with personalization of events being common, or presenting with beliefs that he or she is being spoken about by others or on radio, TV, or in musical lyrics (delusions of reference). The episode leading to presentation may be quite florid with thought disorder, hallucinations, and paranoia, but often this settles to leave a residuum of negative symptoms. Understandably, families and other caregivers can become very concerned about such symptoms and the dis-

TABLE 1.2. **Features of Sensitivity Psychosis**

- Often relatively solitary or shy.
- Gradual onset in teens or /early 20s.
- Relatively minor stress (e.g., leaving home for college, starting work) precipitates episodes.
- Caregivers usually very involved.
  —High expectations (based often on client's past perform ance)
  —Encouraging and supportive
  —May be "trying too hard"
- Feels under pressure but at a standstill.
- Ideas/delusions of reference and thought broadcasting especially frequent—particularly when overstimulated.
- Prominent "negative" symptoms.

abling effect they have, and tend to try very hard to help the person. These efforts, however, can be counterproductive (as discussed in Chapter 12).

CASE 1: GORDON

Gordon, a quiet young man of 18, was referred to see a psychiatrist, presenting with depression after leaving school. He was living with his father, a recently retired attorney, age 66, and his mother, a teacher, age 57. His brother, a police officer, age 24, was described as having "effectively dropped out of school" and now lived in a city 70 miles away with his girlfriend. He knew of no family history of mental illness. He experienced no developmental problems and after going to a local primary school went away to private secondary school as a boarding resident at age 12. He was happy for the first 4 years and did well at his initial public examinations, then started more advanced studies in chemistry, physics, and psychology.

He returned to school after the first year of these studies and felt that he "didn't fit in." He said that he couldn't communicate with the other students, he was ruminating about them, and that their background was more privileged. When he initially became depressed, he had trouble going to sleep. He described "analyzing people's lifestyle and background." He felt inadequate, considered suicide, and indeed deliberately walked over railway bridges, thinking of throwing himself off. He felt he was "in tune with others' thoughts"—that he "could pick them up." He was referred by the school to see a psychologist, who noted his "great difficulty functioning in terms of motivation," but Gordon did not disclose his psychotic symptoms.

He began to experience visual hallucinations of colorful patterns and felt in some way that he was "able to detect other people's characteristics through these patterns." He also began to hear female voices criticizing him. He could not continue at school and left to live at home, where he undertook a local college course in media studies. He remembers that he felt that he "got on well with other students" but had problems with the academic work. He used cannabis occasionally from the age of 16 but not during the 6 months prior to psychiatric referral.

When seen for psychiatric examination he was noted to be spontaneous, with a "pseudophilosophical quality" to his speech, and expressed openly the belief that he was picking up people's thoughts by the characteristics of their voices. He was also considered to be showing blunting of affect and, with his difficulties with work, lowering of motivation, that is, the possible emergence of negative symptoms. This was considered by the psychiatrist assessing him as likely to be a poor prognostic factor.

His parents were seen and disclosed that a paternal uncle had died of suicide 25 years earlier. They described Gordon as previously strong, determined, and thoughtful. However, over the preceding 2 years, he had become increasingly introspective, distant, and irritable, and complained about hearing voices to his mother. His father expressed a very negative view of psychiatric care but was concerned about his son. Medication was commenced—chlorpromazine. He was at this stage referred for cognitive therapy to the psychosis service in Southampton for psychiatric and therapeutic intervention.

He was seen over the next few months as an outpatient. He was noted to be becoming depressed, particularly exacerbated by an incident where he had a minor car accident when driving. His father became very critical, harshly blaming him for the accident, and the home atmosphere became very tense. He was prescribed an antidepressant but discontinued chlorpromazine, an antipsychotic that he had agreed to take. He was continuing at the local junior college, and initially his results were quite good, although he was quite negative about them. His plan was to apply to a 4-year university. However he was going to bed in the early hours of the morning and getting up late, meaning that he was missing lectures.

After a summer vacation he began to miss appointments and his classes. When questioned he said that he had decided to take a year off, but then he changed his mind. His friends had almost all moved away, and so he was seeing them only occasionally and beginning to shut himself off from the world. He missed a few more appointments, and then his family doctor re-referred him, as his parents said that he was refusing to see anyone. His mood was "strange, with inappropriate thoughts and ideas." Fortunately he came to the next interview, being persuaded by his brother and mother. He described serious difficulty completing work at college: "It seems whatever I am thinking about, they can hear my thoughts or know what I am thinking about." He restarted medication, "which helped clear the jumble out," and then dropped out of college altogether for a while. He was confining himself to his room when not taking medication, and his "parents [were] at the end of their tether." He did continue intermittently at college but got very poor grades. He was actively hallucinating, hearing sarcastic comments.

Following the assessment above, we developed a model of his symptoms based on the idea of "sensory overload" that prevented him from functioning; he agreed to take an antipsychotic drug, risperidone, in the morning as a way of "buffering against this stress." His parents were seen together, and the model of negative symptoms was described (see Chapter 12). It was agreed that the best way forward was to reduce pressure and expectation—aim to convalesce. All agreed that he should "take a year off." His mood immediately improved. He still had the "feeling of waves of energy between people" and "I still think I can hear myself thinking out loud and others thinking out loud" (thought echo/broadcasting) with occasional voices. He had not been claiming welfare benefits, so this was initiated.

Over the next few months, he met with the therapist and chatted, working on understanding the thought broadcasting and also "made actions"—deliberately diverting his eyes, which he felt were out of his control but which increased with stress. His father "backed off," and his mother remained supportive, although occasionally she became the subject of Gordon's verbal frustration. His brother visited occasionally and after a few months took him to a rock festival, which was a severe test of his ability to cope with the thought broadcasting, which increased even with small crowds. He also visited other events, for example, the local boat show.

Gordon then decided that he was ready to visit the local job center to make an appointment to see the Disability Resettlement Officer, who could offer him support in looking for suitable meaningful employment. This took a number of weeks of discussing exactly where he needed to go, what he needed to do, and to judge when he felt able to cope with this. Having made the appointment, on leaving the center, he believed that a couple of young men across the road knew what he was thinking and were laughing at him. Fortunately he could talk objectively about this, although he retained a strong degree of conviction that this was what occurred; he was prepared to go to the interview that was eventually scheduled for him, and he attended. This subsequently led to his being offered a place in a residential course on computer programming for a month, which he successfully completed. Since then, he has started part-time work in an office of a friend of his mother's. He is gradually becoming less isolated and is cautiously making progress, as described later in this manual.

Drug-Related Psychosis

The key diagnostic factor with drug-related psychosis is that the first occurrence of psychotic symptoms coincided directly with taking a hallucinogenic drug (see Table 1.3). Cocaine, amphetamines, or ecstasy seem the most common, but high levels of cannabis may also have this effect. Continual use of these drugs may produce further episodes but over time the psychotic symptoms may occur independently of drug usage and other events (e.g., a TV program about drugs or meeting an old friend can cause it, or

---

TABLE 1.3. **Features of Drug-Related Psychosis**

- Drug-induced psychosis at initial presentation (hallucinogens—amphetamine, cocaine, LSD, heavy use of cannabis).
- Recurrence or perpetuation of symptoms when drugs not present (on testing).
- Initially may be given diagnosis of personality disorder or drug misuse (only).
- Hallucinations/paranoia—replay of original psychosis.
- Onset usually in teens or 20s.
- May have "rebellious" personality.
- Frequently from a disrupted family.
- Caregiver often very uncertain how to help and may therefore give confused messages to client.
- Frequently poor cooperation with services.

---

the symptoms may simply persist in the absence of any hallucinogen). This can occur following only one episode of drug-precipitated psychosis. Persistence of symptoms may develop but can readily be tracked back to the initial drug-taking experience. These symptoms tend to be a replay of the original psychosis, at least in part. Work with families and other caregivers is necessary and needs to emphasize consistency, but it may prove difficult as they are often having to deal with quite chaotic and sometimes hostile behavior. Gaining the client's cooperation for treatment, at least during the earliest stage of involvement, can be a major problem.

CASE 2: CRAIG

Craig, a tall, athletic young man with long hair, presented with symptoms that he described as "flashbacks" occurring twice a week. He had suicidal ideation and behavior and had recently taken a large overdose of medication but was fortunately found before serious damage was done. He also was frequently banging his head in response to voices and had considered hanging himself with a wire flex.

He was born in a countryside village. He has two older brothers and a mother who was said to have been unable to cope with them after his birth. She seems to have suffered from postnatal depression, so Craig spent a lot of time with his grandparents. His parents split up when he was 8, and he moved to Nottingham to live with his father, although he continued to have holidays with his mother. He describes a happy childhood despite this and relates well to his family. He did well academically at school up to the age of 17, gaining good passes in basic examinations and commencing advanced studies despite having developed positive signs of schizophrenia. He has no relevant medical history.

He commenced taking cannabis at age 14, followed by LSD and occasional use of heroin. He says that he has generally avoided illicit drugs since developing his illness but remains occasionally vulnerable to friends' influence. He had a number of girlfriends before becoming ill. He has not worked except for assisting his father occasionally.

He presented at age 17 with a 2- to 3-month history of voices, described as seeming to be outside of his head. They sometimes would repeat his thoughts or tell him to do things, including kill himself. He described being made to move in response to them and that his thoughts were withdrawn and possibly broadcast. He developed ideas that he was controlled by a foreign agency and occupied by two people who were influenced in some uncertain way by electronic fields. At the time of presentation he said that he had had no heroin or LSD for 4 months and no cannabis for 2 months. He was prescribed sulpiride, an antipsychotic, and improved over the next few months. He started college but had persistent thought broadcasting and described significant perplexity. He stopped medication because of sedation and started experiencing additionally thought insertion, somatic delusions, and audible thoughts. However, he continued attending college and got a part-time job. He was seen psychiatrically again because he had broken a television and compact disc player in response to voices. Risperidone was used, but he showed erratic compliance.

He was admitted to the hospital after being aggressive toward his brothers and threatening his father with a knife. He took an overdose and tried to hang himself but fortunately was found before coming to serious harm. He also hit his 6-year-old sister in response to voices. He soon settled down in the hospital with medication, however. He then left the hospital and moved out of his father's house to live with friends but then started missing college since he was not getting up early enough. A few weeks later, he smashed a tape recorder and then fell through a window, possibly intoxicated with illicit drugs. His care coordinator arranged with him to move to a group home, and he agreed to see a psychologist but then changed his mind and again took an overdose.

Craig was readmitted to the hospital: he believed aliens were talking to him, telling him to kill himself or his friends. He said he believed the prescribed medication was cyanide and continued to have thought insertion and withdrawal. He improved in the hospital and left to live at a girlfriend's house, but this soon broke down and he went into another supported group home for a few months. He then had a period of 2 years living independently in a flat but became vulnerable to drug-using friends. A further admission occurred due to relapse from the use of illicit drugs and discontinuing antipsychotic medication. He was shouting, irritable, and unable to deal with an accidental fire in his room, causing concern for his safety. He also had delusions of reference about the television, so he had stopped watching it. He was hearing voices and had low mood with suicidal thoughts.

In the hospital, he started depot medication and was discharged to the group home again. He returned to college, but his father soon detected continuing illicit drug use. He became severely thought-disordered, and he was now also drinking heavily. Clozapine was offered, but he refused to continue it after feeling "pole axed" (severely sedated) when he commenced it and has refused to take it since. A fourth brief admission occurred because of friends "bullying" him. He was apprehended while running and screaming with a screwdriver in hand, making threats to his neighbors. There was a report of him using "crack" cocaine by a neighbor. He also threatened to burn his house down. On admission, however, a drug screen was negative. He abruptly left the hospital but was returned to it—he would not participate in a rehabilitation program, so he returned to the group home. Further admission was subsequently necessary after a serious and very large overdose, which interrupted his planned move into a more independent accommodation. Again, his drug screen was negative for illicit drugs. It was at this point that he was referred for engagement in cognitive therapy.

Over a period of 6 months, a formulation has been developed with him looking at the circumstances in which he developed symptoms and when he has relapsed. This has been done in an exploratory and nonjudgmental way, reviewing the reasons for taking illicit drugs as well as the problems they have caused. Attribution of current symptoms to these previous drug-induced episodes has been gradually accepted, and further work on them had been done, as described in subsequent chapters.

Traumatic Psychosis

Posttraumatic stress psychosis (traumatic psychosis) is on a continuum with borderline personality disorder (BPD) and posttraumatic stress disorder (PTSD). Traumatic events—especially sexual abuse in childhood or early adulthood—seem relevant to the symptoms produced (see Table 1.4). For example, the voice may be that of the abuser or, where termination of pregnancy has occurred, of the "unborn child." These become psychotic symptoms because they are externalized by the person and attributed to external agencies, as opposed to PTSD or BPD, where they are recognized as phenomena originating from within. Diagnostic psychotic features such as thought broadcasting and paranoia also occur such that a diagnosis of schizophrenia is warranted. However, work with these clients has to embrace both psychotic symptoms (e.g., understanding voices) and work with borderline features (e.g., impulsivity, fear of abandonment and self-harm, or posttraumatic stress).

CASE 3: GILLIAN

Gillian presented first to general adult psychiatric services at 31 years of age. She was admitted from the family home involuntarily, under the U.K. Mental Health Act, with the help of the police. At that time Gillian was dressed in a garish manner with excessive jewelry, very brightly colored and inappropriate clothing, and heavy makeup. She made reference to a "bionic arm" that was causing her problems at home. Examination revealed that she had severe alopecia (hair loss) due to repeated hair washing and bilateral conjunctivitis due to excessive application of mascara. There was evidence of affective incongruity and preoccupation with personal cleanliness. She appeared to be continually disturbed by auditory hallucinations. Although extremely distressed and extremely mentally unwell, she was deemed to be at low risk of suicide or of violence to others. There was evidence of increasing deterioration in her physical state due to the degree of psychotic preoccupation.

Gillian had a normal birth and development in childhood, though she gradually fell behind her colleagues in elementary school and needed one-to-one instruction. Despite this, she did poorly in examinations, and an educational psychologist made a diagnosis of borderline learning disability. Gillian spent almost all her time with her family. Her father was disabled with rheumatoid arthritis, and Gillian spent a lot of time caring for him up until the time of his premature death when she was only 22 years old. Gillian's mother was a dominating figure who held the family together after her husband's death and used to do the various

---

TABLE 1.4. **Features of Traumatic Psychosis**

- Auditory hallucinations
  —Abusive, violent and/or sexual content
  —Second person ("you're a [swear word]")
  —Command ("Kill yourself," "kill your children")
- Experienced as shocking and alien
- Repetitive and distressing
- Fluctuating insight
- Blames self
- Associated with
  —PTSD, especially sexual abuse
  —Depression; suicidal and depressive thoughts
- Overlap with borderline personality disorder

household chores with Gillian's help. Gillian and her mother were inseparable up until the time of the mother's sudden death of myocardial infarction when Gillian was 29 years of age. By the time of the mother's death the two brothers and two sisters had married and were living away from the family home. This left Gillian alone at home with Jack, the eldest of the brothers, who was a heavy user of alcohol. Jack's friends, who visited the house for drinking sessions, behaved indecently toward Gillian and left money with Jack. Jack bought jewelry and inappropriate clothing for Gillian and coerced her into wearing makeup when his drinking friends were coming to the house. Gillian was effectively used as a prostitute and repeatedly sexually assaulted. Initially she became anxious and depressed with obsessional thoughts and rituals. This rapidly led on to the development of pseudohallucinations and increasing social withdrawal.

By the time she was seen by psychiatric services, Gillian was suffering from virtually continuous auditory hallucinations. These were second-person and command in type. Content included "You are useless," "Put the makeup on," "Don't you have any better clothes?," "You are a slut," and "You are dirty—wash your hair." Gillian believed that the voices were telling the truth but did not know what they were exactly. She reported visual images and at times visual hallucinations linked to the voice-hearing experience.

Gillian derived some benefit from antipsychotic medication, but the hallucinations and negative symptoms were little affected. Assessment revealed that, when prompted, Gillian was quite capable of undertaking a variety of tasks. She was referred for cognitive therapy with a diagnosis of schizophrenia due to failure of response to standard treatment including antipsychotic medication, occupational therapy, and supportive nursing. It was decided first of all to undertake a trial of clozapine for 6 months along with placement in a rehabilitation hostel. Behavioral therapy was used during this period in an attempt to cut down on her repeated hair washing and application of makeup. There was some evidence of minimal improvement on this regime, but at the next review it was decided that cognitive therapy should be attempted to see if Gillian could be more effectively engaged in working with her symptoms on the basis of a mutually understood formulation. Work done with her and her progress are described later in this manual.

Anxiety Psychosis

When anxiety (and, sometimes, depression) increases, often it is in response to stressful circumstances, although these are frequently not recognized as such (see Table 1.5). A "delusional mood" may develop—that is, a feeling that something significant is going to happen that may seem spiritual, magical, or parapsychological. Then a point is reached, often quite abruptly, when the person "knows" the answer that explains what has been happening to them—why they feel the way they do. Often they are isolated and unable to check out such concerns with anybody they trust and whose views they respect. "It is because I am being poisoned by my neighbors—they've never liked me" or "It is because I am descended from the Queen of Scotland and they are all jealous of me." There may then be other symptoms that develop consequent to this, but the key presenting issue is a very strongly held belief for which evidence is lacking—although

TABLE 1.5. Features of Anxiety Psychosis

- Onset
  —Acute: it builds up over a few days or weeks
  —Generally later in life: late 20s onward
- Stress-related (e.g., work pressure)
- Anxiety relieved by crystallization into a "meaningful" explanation for distressing feelings
  —Delusional perception or delusional conclusion (e.g., "the neighbors are responsible" or "I'm persecuted because I've been sent to save them")
- Isolation common
  —Geographic (e.g., living alone or working away from home)
  —Interpersonal (e.g., relationships broken down)
- Usually delusions present—may be grandiose or persecutory—developing into a delusional system
- Further episodes in response to stress

there may be features of the belief that in themselves are true or at least understandable but do not fully support the conclusion that is so strongly held.

CASE 4: PAUL

Paul was seen at home at the request of his family doctor on an urgent basis. At that time he was 28 years old. His parents, one a judge and the other a barrister, were very concerned about his deterioration over the preceding 10 days. They noted that he seemed to be a bit upset a few weeks earlier after finding out that his ex-girlfriend had just become engaged to be married. Thereafter he had struggled, applying for jobs with very little success. He had a degree in fine art that had not opened up the job market for him as he had hoped it might.

Despite these problems, he had seemed quite well until 10 days before the referral. At that point his elder brother had informed the family that he had been promoted to the board of directors of an electronics company. This appeared to have triggered an anxiety reaction in Paul, which led to increasing insomnia and preoccupation. For the 72 hours before his referral he was reported to be extremely anxious, with palpitations, abdominal churning, and tremor. He became increasingly pale, guarded, thought-disordered, and perplexed, culminating in a period of virtually total insomnia for 48 hours. He reported the belief that he might be changing sex on the basis that he had previously enjoyed dressing in women's clothes.

There was no history of substance misuse, and there was no family history of mental illness of any kind. There had been no birth trauma or any developmental problems, but his younger brother (Robert) had been taken into care as a baby when Paul was only 3 years old. He said that this was "a dark family secret which nobody ever talked about." Paul had performed reasonably well at high school and then at college.

After admission to the psychiatric unit he reported that a videotape had been made of him when he was cross dressing in a shop and that he believed that the tape was going to be used to harm him in some way. As his agitation gradually settled, he reported the belief that he was turning into a woman and indicated that the tape had contained material predating the massacre at Dunblane (an incident where a number of children at a school had been shot a few months before), which he believed had put the idea of committing the murders into the mind of the murderer. Consequently he believed that he was to blame for the deaths of the children and that he would shortly be arrested by the police and thereafter incarcerated and vilified. He also believed that he had written some successful popular songs that had been stolen by the artist in question, who had somehow heard the contents of the tape.

His delusional system proved impervious to antipsychotic medication, although his behavior would have been unmanageable without it. There was concern that he may have decided to attempt suicide—such was his degree of distress over the impending "prosecution" that he was convinced was going to occur. On medication his thought disorder, perplexity, and severe somatic anxiety symptoms had all settled, but the delusional system dominated his lifestyle to such a degree as to make his quality of life very poor indeed. In this setting of a treatment-resistant systematized delusion with concerns over suicide risk he was referred for cognitive therapy.

Other Possible Subgroups

There may be other clinical groups, but generally people with a broad diagnosis of schizophrenia seem to fit into the foregoing categories—although some may possibly meet criteria for more than one category. We find them useful in considering management and also as terms that are often much more acceptable than "schizophrenia"—because they are more complete or accurate descriptions of their problems. "Psychosis" as a term can sometimes be troublesome to people—it can be seen as stigmatizing—but replacing it with "disorder" or "problem" (e.g., sensitivity disorder or severe anxiety disorder) is often an acceptable alternative to people experiencing these problems. Negotiating the language we use with people can improve communication, engagement, and eventually shared understanding.

Possible mechanisms for the development of the subgroups are illustrated in Figure 1.1. For each group, there would be expected to be differences in vulnerabilities and stressors that will also influence whether the person develops schizophrenia or other disorders such as depression, borderline personality disorder, or drug dependence, or no disorder at all. Stigmatization will have an amplifying effect, and a tendency toward an externalizing bias (attributing experiences, e.g., voices or things being experienced by the person, to others), which defines psychosis, will need to be present.

UNDERSTANDING SYMPTOMS OF SCHIZOPHRENIA

Symptoms of schizophrenia have been described by influential psychopathologists such as Jaspers (1963) as "nonunderstandable"; however, much experience and research since that time has made them much more understandable. The cognitive model developed to understand delusions, hallucinations, thought disorder, and negative symptoms is discussed here (summarized in Figure 1.2). Part of the process of developing a formulation of a case involves developing a case-specific understanding of the causes, function, meaning, and factors maintaining symptoms.

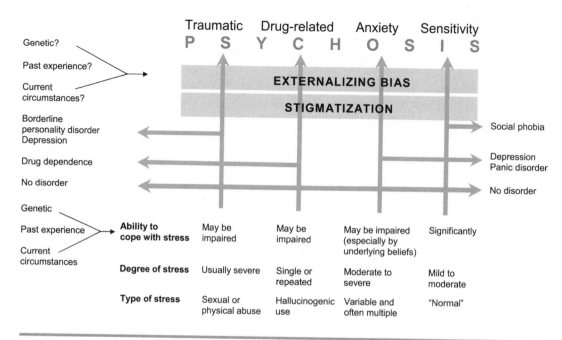

FIGURE 1.1. Theoretical model of subgroups.

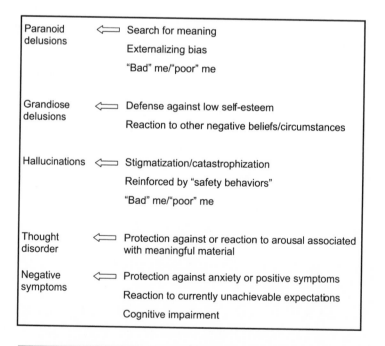

FIGURE 1.2. Symptomatic explanations.

Delusions

Delusional beliefs are the core of psychotic symptoms, including hallucinations, as it is the beliefs about voices, visions, and the like that are fundamentally important rather than the experience of the phenomena themselves (see below). Similarly, thought interference and passivity (dealt with in Chapter 11) are special types of delusion. The term "delusion" is used as a shorthand term for strongly held beliefs that distress the person or interfere with his or her life by affecting important relationships with others. In addition, traditionally, it describes beliefs that are inaccurate, irrational, not amenable to reason, and inconsistent with the individual's culture. We would contend that categorical assumptions of inaccuracy, irrationality, and cultural inconsistency about these beliefs are problematic. In this manual we do not assume that strong beliefs, however strange they may seem, are inaccurate, nor that they need to be changed—but that they need to be understood and their consequences explored. One example where this was relevant involved a woman who had been admitted to the hospital with paranoid "delusions." These were centered around her husband, who she accused of trying to kill her. Her family disputed this, and her husband presented plausibly and appeared very concerned about her. She eventually accepted medication and returned home—only to be admitted to a general hospital a few months later as a result of her general practitioner's concerns. Investigation showed that she was indeed being poisoned. Her husband was arrested and later convicted of attempted murder. While such circumstances are rare, much more commonly bizarre or apparently erroneous beliefs are found to have some truth in them—or at least the reasons why the person believed them to be true become clearer as assessment and therapy progress.

Key elements in assessing and understanding delusions involve:

- *Strength*: How strongly is a belief held?
- *Context*: How unrelated is it to the person's situation?
- *Preoccupation*: How much time does the person spend thinking about the experience?
- *Plausibility*: How understandable is the belief?
- *Personalization*: How much does the person relate an experience to him- or herself?

The reasons for the development of delusions are multiple, and the reasons for the development of any strongly held beliefs apply. For example, such delusions may explain situations or relationships that are confusing to the person and give order and meaning to his or her life. They would be expected to be consistent with beliefs about the self. Social and cultural considerations may be very strong influences—the need to be accepted by family and peers may influence beliefs. It may be that grandiose beliefs in relation to the self (e.g., of special powers or position, such as royalty or divinity) compensate for a perception of lack of respect and a consequent need to impress (but this has yet to be effectively demonstrated). Paranoid beliefs may be related to a particular mood (e.g., depression), which they commonly accompany. They may explain circumstances (e.g., the loss of a job) that seem unfair and possibly allow the person an alternative explanation to one that attributes responsibility for the event that person (e.g., missed time from work), or to chance circumstances (e.g., the person's area of expertise was no longer needed due to a change in market conditions).

Most important is that the formulation of the person's circumstances and symptoms, especially focusing on the initial episode, usually provides ways of finding meaning in delusional beliefs—especially where these are fixed and few in number or part of a delusional system. On occasion, delusions may be presented that are transient and held with less conviction, especially in cases where someone is highly psychotic. These may be less meaningful, but even these often reflect the current and past experiences of the person.

Hallucinations

The cognitive model conceptualizes hallucinations as the person's own thoughts—which, to them, seem to come from *outside* their mind. The relevant belief is therefore that internal thoughts are externally generated phenomena. Traditionally they have been defined as vivid experiences with the quality of external reality in the absence of a stimulus to the sensory apparatus. Auditory, visual, and somatic hallucinations are therefore entirely internal cognitive phenomena that elicit powerful affective and behavioral responses, as they have all the implications of externally valid events. The beliefs about the hallucinations are fundamental. If the person does not recognize that the thoughts emerge from his or her mind—as is quite natural, given the convincing nature of the experience—this can be confusing and often distressing. One aim in developing "insight" will usually be to help the person explore alternatives to this belief.

Voices, the most common presentation of hallucinations, usually present as aversive phenomena: the person is distressed by them. It is widely assumed that voices are pathological—not just by psychiatrists and other mental health workers but especially by the general public. As has become clearer through the work of Marius Romme (Romme & Escher, 1989) and subsequently the "Hearing Voices Network," this is frequently, at best, a simplistic understanding of them and, at worst, an erroneous one. They have shown that many people hear voices that they value and view positively. For example, one rather isolated client heard the voices of two women chatting with him that he described as being very good company. Others may be ambivalent about them—the voices may at times have positive and at other times negative attributes. Certainly those who present to mental health services are more likely to experience negative effects, but even then positive effects can still exist. It is important to understand the impact of voices on the person and their view of them rather than assuming that they are wholly negative. This is so even where the presenting symptoms are abusive, unpleasant voices. Sometimes as voices recede, clients speak of increased loneliness and emptiness because so much of their time was previously occupied with combating them. While this would not usually be a reason for not working with the voices, it is an issue that deserves to be addressed in its own right.

Many people experience functional hallucinations in which the hallucinatory experience tends to be triggered by other perceptions. An example of this would be the person who developed accusatory auditory hallucinations when traffic noise became louder during the rush-hour period. In this case, it was agreed that the main caregiver would call a local window installer to have double glazing installed. The result was extremely effective. Such simple environmental interventions may not be considered be-

cause mental health professionals often do not consider such symptoms ever to be amenable to such simple measures. Assessment is limited, and so precipitants such as the
traffic noise are not identified and interventions not suggested or tried. Many people
also hallucinate in the presence of white noise—indistinct background auditory activity. For example, a client developed marked exacerbation of hallucinations when she
heard a humming sound from the flat downstairs: This turned out to be the neighbor's
spin dryer. The neighbor was entirely agreeable to placing some foam rubber under the
base of the dryer to diminish the noise in this case. Such simple maneuvers are often
possible, although usually other measures are also necessary, but if successful, are seen
as positive experiences allowing therapy to proceed. They encourage the person to further engage with their voice-hearing experience—focus on and work with it—and to
further their understanding and range of coping skills. The person may not engage
with the voices in such a constructive manner without a lead from the mental health
professional. Engagement with the psychotic symptoms by the psychiatrist, psychologist, psychiatric nurse, occupational therapist, or social worker will often allow the person to emerge from stigmatized withdrawal and begin to take some control over the experiences.

Hallucinations are interesting cognitively, both in terms of their form and their
content. In terms of form, the diagnostic hallucinations of schizophrenia are third-
person hallucinations, a running commentary on the person's actions, and a thought
echo. Such symptoms often are "replays" of situations that have occurred or statements
that have been made—usually in distressing or stressful circumstances (third-person
voices and running commentary can resemble family discussions, e.g., "He's not very
good, you know." "He's walking out of the house again"; thought echo is the person's
own thoughts—but externalized). They would also appear to be very similar in type to
the symptoms of obsessive–compulsive disorder (note the similarities and contrasts in
the definition of obsessions, below).

A definition of obsessions (as contrasted with hallucinations)
- Ideas, thoughts, or images that are involuntarily produced (*as are hallucinations*)
- Occurring recurrently and persistently and experienced as senseless and repug-
  nant (*as are some hallucinations*)
- Recognized as products of the person's own minds (*unlike hallucinations*)

Third-person hallucinations involve the same themes as obsessional thoughts (violence, control, religion, sexuality, cleanliness). This may involve the need to resist such
themes by psychologically disowning them. The running commentary could be seen
sometimes as an extension of obsessional indecision and thought echo of the obsessional fear that others will be able to detect the person's unsavory thoughts.

The failure to recognize hallucinations as one's own thoughts defines the difference between obsessions and hallucinations, although in practice these represent a continuum. This group of hallucinations therefore has overlap with obsessions and could
be seen as lying on a spectrum with the symptoms of obsessive–compulsive disorder. If
this is the case, then we might expect normalizing, exposure techniques, and work with
linked schemas (e.g., control, responsibility, the thought–action link, and perfectionism)
to be useful. These are techniques that are often used in working with hallucinations in
schizophrenia.

Some hallucinations in schizophrenia do not have diagnostic implications, although occurring commonly. Examples include second-person and command hallucinations. These are often linked to visual imagery and at times to visual hallucination. These would appear to be a separate group of hallucinatory experiences that are commonly found in the setting of trauma. In the case of women who experience hallucinations long-term, around two-thirds have described having been sexually assaulted. These hallucinations are usually demeaning and derogatory and often comment on the worthlessness of the person or on sexual matters (often alleging homosexuality, pedophilia, or prostitution) and commanding actions usually of self-harm. The voice often resembles that of the abuser, and there can be linked somatic hallucinations (feelings of being touched, often intimately) and olfactory hallucinations (associated smells). In such instances, the hallucinations are usually best conceptualized and discussed as forms of flashback. The linked feeling is often of overarousal or varying degrees of distress and depression. In such cases the diagnosis of an emotionally unstable ("borderline") personality disorder may also be made—but additionally the person has psychotic symptoms, that is, his or her experiences may include hearing voices or thought interference.

Thought Disorder

Formal thought disorder can be fascinating. It can allow us to explore the richness of language and the remarkable ways in which people can combine components to form new words and expressions—and it can also get both you and the person who is talking to you quite frustrated. The content of thought-disordered speech may be quite poetic in nature or simply garbled and seemingly nonsensical.

Essentially, the cognitive model of thought disorder views the term itself as a misnomer—what usually presents to us is not thoughts directly but speech that is idiosyncratic. Not "thought disorder" but communications disorder. Often the person is striving to communicate but hardly managing to. The thoughts (or at least what they are trying to convey) beneath the conversation may be quite logical (once they can be understood), but their expression seems not to be. The person may speak very rapidly, with interweaving themes, using words that most people use with quite different meanings or words that are derived from others—either with unusual grammatical rules attached or as composite words made up of parts or the whole of words used in usual conversation. So, often people—family or staff—give up on them or humor them; this may mean that over the years they will receive little guidance or feedback to assist them in modifying, and thus clarifying, what they mean. They may appear, conversely, not to communicate much at all, or repetitively—with "poverty of content," as it is described. This may be a lack of thoughts or it may be demoralization or simply a lack of much to say because of their social circumstances and the poverty of the environment around them.

People with active thought disorder, including knight's-move thinking (that is, jumping around with just a tenuous connection—as a knight does in chess), fusion of themes, and neologisms (newly created words), are usually highly aroused by specific concerns (Harrow & Prosen, 1978). But they may have significant problems in discussing these issues and as they come closer to discussing them and become more agitated, so the thought disorder becomes greater and greater, interfering with communication. Proceeding slowly and patiently can help in clarification. There may be one core theme that drives the disorganization of thought, and if the person can be helped to focus on this, using thought linkage and explanation, increased coherence can result. By repeatedly but gently asking the person how he or she got from X to Z, the person begins to explain the Y connecting them together. Similarly, neologisms are questioned during speech, and explanations are requested. The underlying driving theme is usually one of threat, fear, or distress, and once this is identified a focus on relevant events and beliefs allows a reduction in arousal and increased coherence of speech. The underlying perceived dangers and threats have often been misperceived or magnified and can be gradually corrected during therapy (Turkington & Kingdon, 1991).

Negative Symptoms

The term "negative symptoms" itself is disheartening, even though it is superficially accurate. What sort of symptoms are they? They are intended to describe absence—of expression, drive, emotion, and thought. But appearances, as elsewhere, may be deceptive. Under the surface, much may be happening in terms of contemplation and observation. Releasing the energy and potential that may be present but suppressed is an essential goal of treatment. All these symptoms have cognitive or behavioral components and so potentially are amenable to cognitive-behavioral approaches. Assessing them accurately assists in the development of a formulation-based treatment plan. Each of these symptoms may be understandable, as follows.

Affective Flattening

The flattening of affect involves difficulty in communicating emotion or expressing feelings through facial expression and tone of voice, but it is worth exploring with the person why he or she appears to have such problems. There are a number of possibilities, but it is wise to find out the individual's own assessment of the issue. You may need to approach the issue sensitively because the person may not have previously realized that this was how he or she was perceived, and it can potentially undermine one's social confidence. As with other symptoms, affective flattening may be biological in origin, in which case striving to change may prove ineffective. However, there are also possible psychosocial factors.

It may be that the person is effectively "in shock." This may be related to past traumatic events that he or she has failed to work though effectively, for example, bereavement. Alternatively, it may be appropriate learned behavior for the circumstances in which the person lived. For example, if shows of emotion (e.g., tears or disagreement) were disapproved of—as is the case in some families and cultures (typified by the British "stiff upper lip")—or punished, or triggered abuse, the absence of reaction—affective flattening—may be a natural reaction. When the early years of the parents of people with schizophrenia, or the persons themselves, have been difficult through poverty or repeated bereavements or other traumatic events, such emotional blunting may be an understandable reaction.

Affective flattening may be a direct reaction to abusive, derogatory voices or thoughts, and the "frozen" expression, a "front" to the world, may be an attempt to cope with seemingly overwhelming disturbance. Depression itself will present with affective flattening as a component of a broad depressive symptomatology. Medication can also contribute. Parkinsonian symptoms can be caused by antipsychotic drugs, especially the older "typical" drugs but also the newer ones in higher doses. These symptoms manifest themselves in a variety of often subtle ways, but reduction in emotional expression is particularly well recognized as a side effect.

Alogia

What is alogia? It is described as slowness to respond, with the amount and content of speech restricted or interrupted. But is this a lack of thoughts or, rather, difficulty in communicating them? How can we know what someone else is thinking? There are suggestions from neuropsychological testing that cognitive deficits may underlie this symptom. But sometimes failure to express may have psychosocial sources. One reaction to criticism, real or perceived, can be to "shut up." Although this may have begun as a reaction to one individual—a teacher or domineering boss or family member—it can generalize and be reinforced by circumstances. Anxiety and perception of pressure certainly can impede communication, causing interruption, even cessation, of thoughts ("thought block"). A couple of embarrassing times when the person "dries up" and is unable to continue can do major damage to confidence and may contribute to apparent alogia.

Avolition

Absence of drive and motivation is possibly the most disabling of symptoms associated with schizophrenia—"My get up and go has got up and gone." It is certainly one of the most frustrating symptoms. The person seems "lazy," "bone-idle," and "never going to get anywhere in life," but perhaps a better description is "driven to a standstill." The effect of stress may impair attention and concentration, and the more effort applied the more pressured the person feels and the worse their attention and concentration become. Impaired attention leads to difficulty in remembering what is said, and when recall is needed, for example, to perform a new task, it cannot be done. Positive symptoms may also develop and worsen matters. Very often it emerges that lack of effort may now seem the problem, but this has certainly not always been the case. People with a wide range of abilities and achievements may present with avolition, but prior attempts at achievement are not usually the issue. A drop-off in performance is common, and a subsequent discussion will often spotlight the failure to achieve the expected results, with additional pressure and anxiety surrounding this. A vicious circle develops in which the more they try, the less able they are to complete tasks successfully, so the more frustrated and demoralized they become; as they repeatedly experience failure, they lose hope for succeeding in the future and gradually try less and less. Others around them may inadvertently contribute by encouragement, which manifests itself as pressure. Society may also increase pressures, for example, to get a job, a partner, and a family. For many people with schizophrenia, this is not an unreasonable long-term goal, but it *is* a short-term nightmare.

For a few people with schizophrenia, getting a job or partner may, however, be unreasonable even long-term, depending on their general functioning—particularly for those with borderline intellectual capacities. If they were slightly less able, they might be excused from such demands, as they would be viewed by those around them as being intellectually, mentally, or learning-disabled. As such they would receive special schooling and other support. In such circumstances, getting a job and the rest would be seen as an achievement in its own right—as a bonus rather than an expectation. However, because some individuals with schizophrenia and limited functioning have managed to struggle through normal schooling, expectations may be unrealistically high. Goals need to be reviewed, one on one, and adjusted on an individual basis.

Anhedonia

What is anhedonia all about? It denotes a feeling of emptiness and reduced interest in activities and relationships. It is differentiated from depression and so is considered a negative symptom rather than primarily an emotional symptom, but such distinctions are not easy to draw. It is not the same as affective flattening, although you would expect an association between the two. It may be related to demoralization, hopelessness, or feeling numbed and because of the potential overlap with depression is viewed by many commentators as not being a *core* negative symptom. Depression, and possibly anhedonia, is very understandable in a disorder with such a stigmatized reputation and one characterized by such distressing and disabling effects.

Attention Deficit

There is certainly good evidence for poor attention and concentration in schizophrenia. Anyone spending more than a few minutes with someone going through an acute episode of schizophrenia will notice that he or she, the therapist, is often functionally alone, with the client's mind elsewhere. Is this due to neuronal interference in the brain? Perhaps—there is certainly good evidence that people with schizophrenia do more poorly on psychometric testing than normal controls. Such reported impairments include effects on executive functioning, attention, global working memory, and spatial working memory. Cognitive impairment predicts long-term outcomes and may be the most important predictor of vocational outcomes. It is also important to take into account the attendant preoccupation with and distraction by hallucinations, especially when these are vivid and intrusive, and also other thoughts, either delusional, obsessional, or simply very worrisome or even interesting, to the person. Certainly if you think the police are coming to get you or the world is ending soon, it is quite likely that your mind will be preoccupied with that rather than therapy, assessment, or psychometric testing. It is possible that the more the person tries to attend, the more overstimulation may contribute to and increase his or her attentional deficit—that is, the more these thoughts about thoughts ("God, aren't I useless") may interfere.

Social Withdrawal

Withdrawal may be a way to cope with overstimulation. Social overstimulation may be a particularly noxious source of stress. Reducing stress or increasing capacity to cope with it may be needed before direct work with the social withdrawal.

The cognitive model of negative symptoms based on these ways of understanding negative symptoms involves consideration of the protective functions that they may have, how they may be a response to currently unachievable expectations, as well as the effects of overstimulation (e.g., concentration difficulties) in a person who may have a biological vulnerability to stress. (This is discussed further in Chapter 12.)

TWO

Evidence for Effective Treatments in Schizophrenia

The evidence relevant to the effective use of pharmacological and cognitive therapy in treating persons with schizophrenia now has a strong foundation. As well as providing a positive support for your own practice, it may be useful to share some of the information given in this chapter with caregivers, the person with schizophrenia, and other clinicians you might work with. The knowledge that effective therapies are now available to assist clients—and the evidence to support such claims—can encourage clients and their families in their search to cope better or even recover from their individual problems.

ANTIPSYCHOTIC MEDICATION

There is strong evidence of the beneficial effects of antipsychotic medication on positive symptoms and on reducing relapse. Since their introduction in the 1950s, drugs like chlorpromazine and haloperidol have transformed the quality of life of many people with psychotic symptoms. These effects are not simply due to sedative effects on agitation but from specific effects of medication on brain receptors and thus on psychotic symptoms. It has become clear with time, however, that there remain a number of people who do not fully respond to medication, especially where negative symptoms are a major problem. Poor insight also often interferes, leading to poor adherence. Side effects also complicate treatment, for example:

- Sedation
- Postural hypotension (a drop in blood pressure on standing)
- Extrapyramidal side effects (tremor, slowness, and rigidity, as in Parkinson's disease)
- Akathisia (restlessness, especially in the legs)
- Tardive dyskinesia (later onset of abnormal involuntary movements, e.g., around the mouth and causing movements of the trunk)

Antipsychotics are effective, to varying degrees, in reducing relapse and the time spent in the hospital but do not alter the course of the disorder. In 1988, one specific drug, clozapine, was shown to have added benefits over that achieved by other antipsychotics (Kane et al., 1988). Clozapine leads to complete remission of symptoms in some cases and to substantial improvement (>20% on overall symptoms) in many more. It also has effects on negative symptoms, suicidal thinking, and depression. Unfortunately, however, it can have a serious effect on white blood cells, which means that regular blood testing is needed, and it has a variety of other side effects as well, including excessive salivation, convulsions, and sedation.

Over the 1990s, a group of new drugs were introduced designed to reproduce the positive effects of clozapine without the side effects: the "atypical" antipsychotics such as risperidone, olanzepine, quetiapine, amisulpride, and ziprasidone. Unfortunately there is little evidence that they have the specific effectiveness of clozapine, but they do have a different side effect profile that is generally better than the earlier antipsychotics (Geddes et al., 2000). These newer antipsychotics may not exacerbate cognitive deficits (as occurs with the older drugs) and may actually improve them. However, they may cause, for example, sedation and weight gain. Weight gain can exacerbate negative symptoms, worsen depression, and lower self-esteem. It may have a role in increasing morbidity and mortality by producing obesity with consequent deleterious effects on health. The generally better side effect profile might also produce improved adherence. Taking medications more regularly and experiencing improved cognitive functioning could well have a synergistic effect with psychological treatments.

FAMILY WORK

Prior to the use of cognitive therapy for individuals with schizophrenia, research into behavioral family interventions flourished in the 1980s. Four independent and methodologically sound studies in the United States and England came up with the same positive conclusions. Leff and colleagues (1985) and Falloon and colleagues (1985) demonstrated the efficacy of modifying high expressed emotion (EE), criticism, or overprotection by caregivers, in preventing relapse at 2-year follow-up (20% in the family work group without medication and 17% with medication, as compared to 78% with medication alone and 83% with no treatment). Hogarty and colleagues (1991) confirmed the benefit of family work and showed no additional improvement with the addition of social skills training. Tarrier and colleagues (1989) again confirmed a positive benefit on relapse and showed no added benefit with the addition of psychoeducation.

In contrast to these findings, McCreadie and Robinson in the Nithsdale study (1987) showed no difference in relapse rates in people living on their own with low-EE or with high-EE relatives. Also, the amount of contact with high-EE relatives did not affect relapse rates. One possible explanation of this finding is that in the Nithsdale study EE was measured when the person was not in a state of relapse, unlike the other studies. It may well be in the Camberwell study (Vaughan & Leff, 1976) that the relapsing person increased the level of EE in the caregivers. One further problem in this area of research was pointed out in the Nithsdale studies (McCreadie & Robinson, 1987). It was very difficult to find enough suitable candidates for family work based on expressed emotion reduction. In this survey 87% of people with schizophrenia were not living in a high-contact/high-EE family. Most of the relatives in this study showed stability in their EE status and only a minority moved between high- and low-EE status. It may be that living with a high-EE relative is associated with relapse but that living with a low-EE relative may protect against it. Nevertheless recent meta-analyses (e.g., Pilling et al., 2002) have concluded that family work is effective in significantly reducing relapse in subgroups of people with schizophrenia, especially those who have high-EE relatives.

In contrast to the family work mentioned so far, which has been essentially cognitive-behavioral, individual psychodynamically informed supportive psychotherapy along with family intervention and deinstitutionalization has been developed in Finland and labeled the "needs-adapted model" (Alanen et al., 1991). Using this approach at 5-year follow-up, 46% of clients had no psychotic symptoms and 29% had worked all of the preceding year (Salokangas et al., 1991). Such a complete change in management practice has not yet been possible in most countries, and replication of the research is needed elsewhere.

COGNITIVE AND BEHAVIOR THERAPY FOR SCHIZOPHRENIA

The development of cognitive therapy in schizophrenia has been based on approaches treating the syndrome of schizophrenia (see Table 2.1) and targeted on individual symptoms such as delusions (Table 2.2) and hallucinations (Table 2.3).

Beck (1952) described a seminal case of a person with a systematized paranoid delusion (probably schizophrenia in DSM-IV-TR terms) treated with a cognitive-behavioral approach with psychodynamic understanding. He described some of the key elements of a new structured psychotherapy of schizophrenia, which, at least in this case, were extremely successful. He engaged with the person and established a working therapeutic alliance in which trust developed. Together they worked on the sequence of events that had preceded the emergence of the systematized paranoid delusion from which the person suffered. A phase of systematic, graded reality testing followed in which the person was guided to examine the evidence in relation to the behavior of his presumed persecutors in a systematic way. He was to attempt to clearly identify his persecutors and then examine and write down their manner of dress, facial expressions, and general behavior and demeanor. Having done this with the help of the therapist in session, he reviewed all the evidence at his disposal from his homework exercises. Eventually, as he felt more confident in his now "safer" environment, he became bolder in examining the behavior of normal people in his community whom he had presumed to be members of a government agency. Gradually he started to eliminate from his suspicions some and finally all of his presumed persecutors. In this case there was no emergence of depression or anxiety as the delusion receded, and the effect appeared to be durable with the person remaining well at follow-up.

However, there was very little further work using this way of working until the late 1980s. At this stage, the lead author was working with a cohort of people with ICD-9 schizophrenia who had either been referred from a catchment area by general practitioners or were already being seen in outpatient clinics, inpatient units, and hostels (Kingdon & Turkington, 1991). All these people were treated using varying degrees of cognitive therapy as well as standard treatment: medication, sheltered accommodation

TABLE 2.1. Use of Cognitive Therapy with Schizophrenia

Authors (year)	Description	Results
Beck (1952)	A successful single-case study with description of techniques and psychodynamic understanding	Diagnosis not given; no use of multiple baselines or any validated measure of change
Meichenbaum & Cameron (1973)	CT improved attentional deficits in schizophrenia	Cohort study, uncontrolled
Kingdon & Turkington (1991, 1994)	The development of improved engagement, using a normalizing rationale	Cohort study, uncontrolled, no symptomatic ratings; theoretical manual
Fowler et al. (1995)	Description of a manual for CT focusing on individual formulation and schema change	Theoretical manual
Kemp et al. (1996)	The development of a brief CT intervention capable of improving adherence with medication	Controlled evaluation
Drury et al. (1996)	Testing of CT in an RCT for the treatment of psychotic relapse. CT seemed to be viable with acutely psychotic inpatients	Significant differences in baseline medication, leading to confounding
Birchwood & Igbal (1998)	The importance of detecting and treating depression in schizophrenia	Theoretical paper
McGorry et al. (1996)	Development of CT delivered during prodrome and first-episode schizophrenia	Uncontrolled evaluation
Kuipers et al. (1997)	RCT in schizophrenia	Beneficial effects. Not blind, fidelity uncertain, treatment as usual control
Tarrier et al. (1998)	RCT in schizophrenia	Positive effects: CT more likely to cause 50% improvement than symptoms counseling. Effects not sustained
Pinto et al. (1999)	RCT showing benefits of CT over and above that of clozapine	Lack of time for clozapine response and underdosing with clozapine
Sensky et al. (2000)	RCT of CT versus "befriending"	Both groups improved over 9 months, continued effect at 18 months for CT
Turkington, Kingdon, et al. (2001, 2002)	General psychiatrists can effectively use cognitive techniques, as can nurses	Small numbers, therapist was highly trained. Large numbers; effect on depression, overall symptoms, and insight
Durham et al. (2002)	RCT with nonspecialist psychologists	Limited but measurable effects
Lewis et al. (2002)	SoCRATES RCT in early schizophrenia	Accelerates improvement in target symptoms but gains lost by 6 weeks
Gumley et al. (2002)	RCT targeting relapse	Positive effect
McGorry et al. (2002)	Prodromal study—6 months CT and risperidone	Delays transition at 6 months, no difference at 1 year
Rector et al. (2003)	Canadian RCT	Benefits for depression and negative symptoms

Note. CT, cognitive therapy; RCT, randomized controlled trial.

TABLE 2.2. **Use of Cognitive Therapy with Delusions**

Authors (year)	Description	Results
Milton et al. (1978)	Study showing belief modification to improve delusions and confrontation to exacerbate delusions	Uncontrolled, cohort study, small numbers
Hole et al. (1979)	A cohort of people with delusions treated with CT with reduction in conviction in most and improvement in other parameters in all	Uncontrolled, cohort study, small numbers
Hemsley & Garety (1986)	Described typical reasoning processes in deluded people	Low numbers of people involved
Fowler & Morley (1989)	Showed improvement in delusions when CT used to analyze the evidence	Uncontrolled cohort study, small numbers
Roberts (1991)	Described how many delusions could be understood in relation to the person's life narrative	Theoretical paper
Turkington et al. (1996)	Described an evidence-based definition of delusion	Theoretical paper
Turkington & Siddle (1998)	CT techniques for delusions described in detail	Theoretical paper

Note. CT, cognitive therapy.

TABLE 2.3. **Use of Cognitive Therapy with Hallucinations**

Authors (year)	Description	Results
Romme & Escher (1989)	Destigmatizing the voice hearer and developing the Hearing Voices network for group support	No studies undertaken
Kingdon & Turkington (1991)	Description of reattribution and work with content of voices	Descriptive with brief cases
Scott et al. (1992)	Description of clear techniques helping hallucinations to change to pseudohallucinations and then obsessional thoughts	Case study with no outcome measures
Chadwick & Birchwood (1994)	Description of the use of working with dysfunctional attitudes (omniscience and omnipotence) in hallucinations	Uncontrolled, adequate sample size, clear methodology
Turkington & Kingdon (1996)	Description of the technique of using rational responding to voice content	Theoretical paper
Haddock et al. (1996)	Focusing versus distraction techniques	Small numbers, nonblind raters, no difference
Morrison (1998)	Description of safety behaviors maintaining some hallucinations	Theoretical paper
Rector & Beck (2002)	A CT model of hallucinations	Theoretical paper

Note. CT, cognitive therapy.

and work, day hospital care and community mental health team support. (A description of the service at the time is given in Groves, 1990). The cognitive therapy approach was acceptable to the group and their caregivers, and for the most part people enjoyed and were keen to attend sessions to discuss their various psychotic symptoms and their causes. There were no suicides or homicides, and the relapse rate was low over a 5-year period. Also, the group were maintained on relatively low-dose antipsychotic medication (mean chlorpromazine equivalent dose = 249.1 mg per day).

At the same time, Tarrier and colleagues (1990) were developing the use of coping skills enhancement (CSE). Also Fowler and Morley (1989) and Chadwick and Lowe (1990) were publishing small cohort case studies. In 1991 Roberts described how delusions could be made more understandable in relation to a person's life history and could even fit in with such a narrative. Tarrier and colleagues (1993) tested their individual psychological treatment for schizophrenia, CSE against problem solving in a randomized controlled trial (RCT) with the target being positive symptom reduction. Problems included a high dropout rate and lack of diagnostic clarity, and the fact that all people who entered the study were analyzed (as they used a "per protocol" methodology). The CSE group showed benefit on the delusion scale of the Psychiatric Assessment Scale (PAS; Krawiecka et al., 1977) and in overall symptom severity on the Brief Psychiatric Rating Scale (BPRS) at the end of therapy and at follow-up. However, despite being a briefer, more intensive, and more focused intervention (10 sessions over 5 weeks) than that of the later studies such as that of the London–East Anglia Study (Kuipers et al., 1997), it had a similar effect size on overall symptoms. Early studies of hallucinations were also being performed showing symptom improvements with both focusing and distraction techniques (Haddock et al., 1996).

Garety and Hemsley (1994) in a controlled pilot study with nonrandom allocation showed that an average of 16 sessions of cognitive therapy was significantly more effective than the control group in reducing delusional conviction, overall symptomatology on the BPRS, and level of depression as measured by the Beck Depression Inventory (BDI; Beck et al., 1961). Drury and colleagues (1996) published a randomized study of cognitive therapy versus supportive counseling in the treatment of acute psychotic relapse. This showed that by the end of 12 weekly sessions the cognitive therapy group was significantly improved in terms of overall symptoms and positive symptoms, particularly delusions. People who had recent onset psychotic symptoms seemed to benefit greatly from direct cognitive therapy work while in the acute ward. Unfortunately, the benefits of the intervention were lost by 5-year follow-up, and the author recommended that booster sessions be used to maintain the effect. Lecompte and Pelc (1996) performed a randomized controlled study that showed an effect size compatible with later studies. The intervention was also shown to be cost-effective.

The London–East Anglia group published initial findings (Kuipers et al., 1997) and followed this up with papers on prediction of outcome (Garety et al., 1997) and cost effectiveness (Kuipers et al., 1998). They showed benefits for cognitive therapy over treatment as usual in the treatment of people with stable psychotic symptoms. The therapists in the study were expert clinical psychologists, and 20 sessions of manualized cognitive therapy were delivered. However raters, though independent, were not blind, and fidelity to the treatment manual as evaluated by an independent rater was not undertaken.

Tarrier and colleagues (1998) in a well-designed methodologically robust study tested cognitive therapy against supportive counseling and routine care. Again they used an intensive approach of two sessions per week over 10 weeks. They used a random allocation design, and the people with schizophrenia entered were broadly representative of the overall population with schizophrenia. The results showed that both cognitive therapy and supportive counseling (SC) were significantly better than treatment as usual (TAU) at 3 months. Cognitive therapy had a significant effect on positive symptoms, whereas SC did not. Significantly more people who received cognitive therapy showed a >50% improvement in positive symptoms. Relapse rate and time spent in the hospital were significantly worse in the TAU group. However the brief intensive therapy of this study was not significantly different from supportive therapy at 1-year follow-up after discontinuation of therapy (Tarrier et al., 1999).

In Italy, Pinto and colleagues (1999) carried out a randomized study of cognitive therapy in people who were beginning treatment with clozapine. Unfortunately the results of the study are difficult to interpret due to the effects of clozapine being variable in terms of time of onset of effect (any time up to 6 months) and a number of people being on subtherapeutic doses due to side effects. Despite these confounding factors the cognitive therapy group showed a significant effect in terms of overall symptoms. Our group (Sensky et al., 2000) compared 9 months of cognitive therapy with befriending (designed to be a control for "nonspecific" therapy factors including time spent with subjects) in a randomized controlled the trial. At end of therapy, both groups had made substantial improvements in depressive, positive, and negative symptoms. In the cognitive therapy group, further gains were made in the subsequent 9 months, while the befriending group scores began to return to their previous levels. Recently Durham and colleagues (2003) have found positive but modest results using a group of cognitive therapy trained therapists who had limited training and supervision in cognitive therapy for psychosis. Gumley and colleagues (2003) have also shown positive benefits on relapse.

Sixteen randomized controlled studies have now been published investigating cognitive therapy for people with schizophrenia. Reviews of these (Dickerson, 2000; Rector & Beck, 2001) and meta-analyses (Gould et al., 2001; Pilling et al., 2002) have confirmed the efficacy of the techniques in people with persistent symptoms for both positive and negative symptoms. These studies have shown benefits at the end of therapy with retention at 6 months to 1 year after completion, in some cases increasing still further. At longer-term follow-up (i.e., more than 1 year after end of therapy), some benefits may be retained but most are lost, suggesting that further "booster" sessions may be necessary. Control interventions designed to control for time and social interaction (e.g., supportive therapy and befriending) tend to have an effect between that of cognitive therapy and treatment as usual. All the interventions in these studies have been additional to the use of medication. This is on the basis that there is strong evidence that antipsychotic medication is effective in both treating symptoms and reducing relapse. Cognitive therapy has been helpful in discussing this evidence and debating the use of medication productively (see Chapter 7). Cognitive therapy can improve collaboration with its usage but does appear to have effects over and above that which could be attributed to improved adherence to medication regimes alone.

The evidence in early schizophrenia is less strong, although small durable benefits were found in the one large study in this area (SoCRATES—Lewis et al., 2002). Studies of the use of cognitive therapy in the prodromal phase (prior to diagnosis of schizophrenia) are currently under way (e.g., Morrison et al., 2002) with one such study showing effects on delaying transition to psychosis in combination with risperidone (McGorry et al., 2002). Both published studies have used relatively brief interventions lasting less than 6 months. During the intervention periods, effects have been seen, but these have been limited in their long-term durability.

There are no studies yet in younger (under 16) or older people (over 60), and there remain issues about whether cognitive therapy for schizophrenia is effective as currently developed cross-culturally (Rathod et al., 2003). One study has shown benefits from using an intervention using motivational interviewing with cognitive therapy for psychosis for people with psychosis and substance misuse (Barrowclough et al., 2001). Research is therefore well advanced, but further areas await exploration.

A summary of the results of these studies would seem to suggest a clear effect on overall symptoms, with some evidence of durability for 20 sessions of cognitive therapy over 6 months to 1 year, delivered by well-trained and supervised therapists. Those receiving therapy have tended to adhere better to antipsychotic medication and to spend fewer days in the hospital when given cognitive therapy. Active control conditions (i.e., supportive counseling and befriending) tended to perform well, with equal benefit to cognitive therapy at short-term follow-up. The interventions appeared to be cost-effective. Results overall seemed well established for delusions and hallucinations and are emerging for negative symptoms.

FIELD STUDIES OF PSYCHOSOCIAL INTERVENTIONS IN SCHIZOPHRENIA

Haddock et al. (1994) noted that community psychiatric nurses were well placed to deliver cognitive therapy interventions in the community. The International Cochrane Collaboration review of cognitive therapy for psychoses (Jones et al., 1999) indicated that the main outstanding question in this area of study was whether the techniques of cognitive therapy that had been delivered with clear evidence of benefit by expert therapists could be delivered in the community by members of community health teams. Field studies have been undertaken with psychoeducation, family intervention, assertive community treatment, intensive case management, and standard case management. This is particularly important as, compared to pharmacological studies, the findings from psychosocial randomized, controlled trials can be much less generalizable due to differences in the quality of the intervention, setting, and participants.

Delivery of psychoeducation in schizophrenia is an important basic skill for community psychiatric nurses. Education can be delivered in the form of training, pamphlets, videos, and group discussion. A review by the International Cochrane Collaboration indicated that there was evidence of psychoeducation in schizophrenia reducing relapse, although the number needed to treat (NNT) was high at 9 (confidence intervals = 6–22) (Pekkala & Merinder, 2000). There is no evidence that psychoeducation can improve adherence to medication, and the mechanism for the effect on relapse has therefore yet to be elucidated.

As previously discussed, family work in schizophrenia targeted on decreasing stress within the family and reducing relapse has proven to be more effective in terms of reducing relapse (NNT = 7, confidence intervals = 4–14). Such family work aims to educate the family about the illness of schizophrenia, improve coping, and facilitate optimal response styles to particular types of symptoms or potential relapse. Targets also include stress management and improved problem solving. High expressed emotion equates to expressions of anger and criticism but also to emotional overinvolvement (often mediated by excessive guilt). Despite the benefits reported by caregivers and in terms of reduced relapse, there is no evidence of reduced burden upon the family.

There is evidence that field studies have failed to replicate the very good results achieved in the early studies where the intervention was delivered by experts. In the case of cognitive therapy, benefits can accrue when delivered in community settings (Turkington et al., 2002). In this study, community nurses who received a brief (2–3 weeks) training and then supervision provided six cognitive therapy sessions for the client and three for the main caregiver (where there was one). Good clinical outcomes were achieved at end of therapy with insight (NNT = 10) and depression (NNT = 9) and further statistically significant improvements with overall symptoms (NNT = 13). In England, the National Institute of Clinical Excellence—a governmental body—has produced guidelines on schizophrenia (National Institute for Clinical Excellence, 2002) that recommend cognitive therapy on an individual basis (at least 10 sessions over at least 6 months) for all those people with residual symptoms of schizophrenia.

THREE

Early Intervention

If someone has a treatable mental health problem, it seems self-evident that this person deserves treatment as early as appropriate to minimize distress and disability. Early intervention may reduce damage to the person's social situation (e.g., loss of job, disturbance to relationships with friends and family) and also to self-esteem. It has also been suggested that there is an "added" value to early intervention in schizophrenia—in other words, that it improves long-term outcomes for clients. Is there a "window of opportunity" to be exploited? Or is there a danger of inappropriate or frankly erroneous labeling, which leads to individuals' becoming distressed and precipitates the outcome feared (i.e., a psychotic illness)? This chapter examines these issues and specific interventions relevant to different presentations. It refers to some topics discussed in later chapters of the book, and readers may find it easier to understand after they have read these later chapters.

Relevant questions are as follows:

- Does early intervention improve prognosis?
- What forms should such intervention take?
- Does early intervention prevent transition to psychosis?
- Is there a correlation between a short duration of untreated psychosis (DUP) and good prognosis?

Most but not all studies do seem to show that improvement in prognosis is positively correlated with early intervention; however, this conclusion is confounded by the fact that short- and long-DUP groups have not been matched. Acute onset is associated with precipitation by easily recognizable life events and with good outcomes, so it can be difficult without long-term randomized controlled studies (which are possibly unethical) to determine whether early intervention improves prognosis.

Services for early intervention in psychosis are being developed internationally (especially in Australia, Scandinavia, and the United Kingdom). These generally incorporate the use of medication and, increasingly, psychological treatment; either each is used alone, or, more commonly, they support each other. Both medication and cognitive therapy have demonstrable effects on established symptoms, but are under-researched in regard to prodromal symptoms (i.e., those symptoms occurring before diagnosis of schizophrenia can be made) and even in early schizophrenia. It could be argued that psychological intervention may be safer, with fewer side effects than medication, and may be less stigmatizing and more acceptable to clients.

So, if nevertheless we decide that early intervention is worth attempting, is it possible? How can we define early symptoms? This has been done in studies (see Table 3.1) where symptoms are either brief, although with significant conviction or severity, or longer in duration but less severe. Can DUP be reduced? There is certainly some recent evidence from Norway, where DUP has been reduced in the target population from 1.5 years to 0.5 years. But how relevant is this to other areas? DUP has been reported as averaging 1 to 2 years internationally, but in the United Kingdom, a large recent study found a mean DUP of 37 weeks and median of 3 months. This therefore means that there is a significant but small number of outliers with very long DUP. Are these different in type from the others?

The evidence that shortening DUP improves prognosis is also limited, although it makes sense that it should do so. Is there evidence of differential benefits of treatment in early compared to late schizophrenia? There is some evidence that pharmacological intervention may be of benefit, but the evidence for cognitive-behavioral therapy is limited. The SoCRATES study (Lewis et al., 2002) suggested that cognitive therapy leads to improved recovery in symptoms early on, compared to routine care alone (in the 5-week intensive therapy period). Effects were small, although measurable and durable, with a dose–response relationship but with no impact on time to relapse (Tarrier et al., 2004).

Can we reduce the rates of transition to psychosis by very early intervention? Again, evidence is limited, although it is emerging through ongoing studies using medication and cognitive-behavioral therapy. In both SoCRATES and a study of 6 months of cognitive therapy and medication in prodromal symptoms (McGorry et al., 2002), effects of cognitive therapy were seen during the therapy period; however, these were then lost after therapy was discontinued, which may suggest that a more sustained period is needed. But there is a question about how relevant early intervention is. It seems that only a minority of people who eventually are given a diagnosis of schizophrenia are detected and offered services by early intervention teams even where these are well

TABLE 3.1. Definition of Prodromal Symptoms in Early Intervention Trials

Brief limited intermittent psychotic symptoms (BLIPS)
- Score > 3 on PANSS delusions or hallucinations
- Score > 4 on PANSS conceptual disorganization
- Lasting more than a week and resolving without antipsychotic medication

Attenuated symptoms
- Score of 3: delusions
- Score of 2–3: hallucinations
- Score of 3–4: cognitive disorganization or suspiciousness

Note. PANSS, Positive and Negative Symptom Scale.

TABLE 3.2. **Early Intervention for Sensitivity Psychosis**

- Alert services that have contact with young people to the need to discuss with mental health services cases where "odd" symptoms are present.
- Ensure that mental health services respond promptly and appropriately.
- Manage any overlap with adolescent crisis.
- Establish a dialogue with the client and his or her family, and provide contact numbers even if no mental illness is diagnosed.
- Identify anxiety and depressive symptoms—normalize, psychoeducate, and use assertiveness and social skills training.
- Reduce individually perceived pressure.
- Assist in learning stress management techniques.

developed with good community contacts. Yet if early intervention is offered—as mental health services and even some governments are now attempting to do—it should be available to as many people as possible who develop symptoms.

The reasons why contact may not be made are not known, but part of the answer may be that these clients:

- Are not "help seekers" and strenuously avoid services.
- Are older or younger than the age groups targeted by teams, which have tended to include just those age 14–35.
- Present with symptoms leading to a diagnosis of affective disorder, puerperal illness, substance misuse, or personality disorder, which only evolves into a diagnosis of schizophrenia after months or even years.

What is clear is that there are many differing presentations, and this is another area where differentiation into subgroups may help with early detection and intervention.

Early intervention services have probably been most effective with, and indeed are usually targeted at, the groups of people whom we have described as having a sensitivity psychosis (see Table 3.2). A whole systems approach is used to identify people presenting with what may be developing psychosis, generally from a position of having been coping reasonably well or at least in a stable position. (Sometimes sensitivity psychosis, however, may arise in persons with, e.g., a learning disability or mild mental retardation.) As people in this group seem to have brief intermittent symptoms as well as low-grade ones, being available when they are having or have just experienced a short-lived episode seems very important. Sometimes the symptoms resolve spontaneously or with minimal intervention, but especially where this is the case, assessment needs to ensure that there are no ongoing stressors (e.g., within the family environment) and, if stressors do exist, that support is offered. Such support (e.g., through family work) may not be accepted, but continuing contact needs to be made—or, at least, a telephone number needs to be obtained, so that contact can be rapidly reestablished.

The issue of how mental health services respond to contacts is also very important. So many families describe how their first contact led to a dismissive discharge on the basis of "adolescent crisis," "personality disorder," or "just substance misuse." Although the evidence at the time may justify such a diagnosis, continuing access to services and an acceptance that these symptoms are common precursors of psychotic illness may reduce the likelihood of closure, rejection, and missed opportunities to provide appropriate support and intervention. Early intervention teams, when available, are in an excellent position to provide this type of assessment and support.

For a person with a sensitivity psychosis, commonly the most important initial management strategy after assessment and formulation is to help the person and his or her family reduce the pressure to which they feel subject. This may mean advising, for example, "taking a year off" from school, work, or college and allowing caregivers to "let go"—that is, to ease off and show their good intentions by supporting and being available rather than asserting strong points of view. This has a beneficial effect on both emerging positive and negative symptoms (see Chapter 12).

Similar tactics are relevant in working with people presenting with drug-induced psychosis (see Table 3.3). Although the initial presentation may be clearly drug-related, in our experience of working in community mental health teams, a majority of those presenting with psychotic symptoms serious enough to warrant contact with mental health services seem to go on to have protracted psychotic illnesses. (The ready availability of substance misuse services may have influenced this view, as those with a long-standing history of substance misuse may have been preferentially referred to such services.) It is therefore important to provide support to the caregivers and to these persons themselves after they have recovered. This can be very frustrating when a person continues to misuse substances, although motivational interviewing may help. But intervention when a person is ready to receive it, and support for caregivers (who can feel very alone and frustrated), can make long-term management much more successful whenever it becomes necessary.

Presentation of traumatic psychosis tends to be quite different, in that the initial diagnosis in such a case is often borderline personality disorder (BPD), puerperal illness, obsessive–compulsive disorder, social phobia, or depressive psychosis, and it is only when clinicians decide that the person has a psychotic illness that the management route changes (see Table 3.4). Alternatively, the person may have been coping relatively well, but then incidents (e.g., within relationships) lead to decompensation and presentation to services. Unfortunately many services working with BPD will not do so if a person is considered to be or becomes "psychotic." Paradoxically, the skills involved in working with reattribution so that BPD work can continue are readily accessible (see especially Chapter 10) and seem to work quite well with this group. Early intervention therefore can mean detecting the tendency to externalize flashbacks or voices and working through therapy to reattribute them to their source—usually traumatic events in earlier life.

TABLE 3.3. **Early Intervention for Drug-Related Psychosis**

- Acute presentation is common.
- Immediate management of acute drug-induced psychosis is recommended.
- Enlist caregivers' support and enhance caregivers' access to services.
- Use cognitive-behavioral therapy reattribute psychotic symptoms to the original episode.
- Undertaken substance misuse management using motivational interviewing.

TABLE 3.4. Early Intervention for Traumatic Psychosis

- Identify relevant events, often many years before.
- Be aware of conditions gradual evolution—the client may initially receive a diagnosis of borderline personality disorder (BPD).
- Therapeutic work with clients who have BPD to reduce externalizing behavior may prevent the progression to psychosis.
- Acute precipitation through stress is possible.
- Reattribution of hallucinations is central to success.
- Work with the power and veracity of voices.
- Deal with key events by discussing client's beliefs and attitudes.
- Then use direct management of BPD (e.g., using dialectical behavioral therapy) may be relevant approach.

Finally, people who develop delusional beliefs abruptly as a result of stressful circumstances—or a gradual increase in anxiety and depression—seem to be a group that could benefit greatly from early intervention (see Table 3.5). The prompt discussion of alternative explanations to the delusional meaning that a client has attributed to feelings or events could potentially reduce the hardening of those beliefs by secondary reinforcement from the reactions of others and simply the effects of time and consolidating behavior by the person. Once a paranoid or grandiose belief emerges, it can be readily reinforced when other people dispute or ridicule it, or avoid the person because of his or her "strange" ways. Normalizing explanations (e.g., about poor sleep and the effects of isolation) can be particularly effective and indeed welcomed.

Initially, these people may present with anxiety or depression and may not even have reached mental health services. Recognition of emerging psychosis—often beginning with statements like "It's as if . . . "—by services, family doctors, or others could allow such intervention to occur. As these people present later in life, early intervention teams targeting individuals under age 35 may miss them, and there is a strong case for teams' extending their remit to this group.

In conclusion, cognitive therapy can be a valuable adjunct to early intervention (see Table 3.6) in the way that it assists identification of psychotic symptoms through its use as a collaborative, exploratory way of working in other mental disorders. It can potentially reduce transition to psychosis by use of reattribution techniques. It can guide the development of early intervention responses from services, and it can be acceptable to clients. In short, it promises to be an effective intervention at this time.

TABLE 3.5. Early Intervention for Anxiety Psychosis

- Rapid engagement and access to services are key elements of success.
- Object is to detect and manage delusional mood in nonpsychotic patients.
- Immediate and consistent work on reattribution is useful.
- Management of associated depressive and anxiety symptoms is a necessary aim.
- Normalize experiences (e.g., suicidal thoughts) and feelings "as if" they were controlled.
- If beliefs or voices are persistent, use inference chains (e.g., "If we did believe you, what would it mean to you?").

**TABLE 3.6. Use of Cognitive Therapy
in Early Intervention**

Valuable as an assessment tool
- Identifying "as if" issues
- Delusional mood
- Incipient passivity—"like being controlled"
- "Perhaps" mechanisms

Role as therapeutic intervention with preventative role
- Using normalization and instilling hope
- Acceptability to the client's group
- Possible to use in limiting transition to psychosis

EARLY INTERVENTION

Gordon (*sensitivity psychosis*): Fortunately, Gordon presented early. He was encouraged by one of his parents to see his general practitioner, who recognized that Gordon was unwell, although he was unsure about exactly what was wrong with him. The doctor asked for a psychiatric opinion, which was offered within a week, and the psychiatrist concluded that psychotic symptoms were present. Coincidentally, a discussion about the use of cognitive therapy in psychosis with the psychiatrist led to Gordon's referral and the rapid involvement of an experienced cognitive therapist. Although this has not prevented further emergence of symptoms, it has probably ameliorated them. Gordon has never required hospitalization and is making good progress.

Craig (*drug-related psychosis*): In contrast, Craig was initially thought correctly to be misusing drugs, but only after a number of contacts with services and much frustration for those around him was he taken on by mental health services; eventually, he was referred to an assertive outreach service. Subsequently, because of the severity and medication-resistant nature of his symptoms, he was referred for cognitive therapy.

Gillian (*traumatic psychosis*): The symptoms that Gillian had were well entrenched by the time she was brought involuntarily into the hospital. She had been ill for at least 6 months, and neglect and abuse during the period prior to this had not been detected. It is difficult to know how earlier intervention could have occurred, although possibly an awareness of her long-standing vulnerability by local health and social services might have allowed action to be taken (and, indeed, protection to be provided) to prevent the development of symptoms.

Paul (*anxiety psychosis*): Intervention in Paul's case was prompt and appropriate; within 10 days of this developing symptoms, he had been assessed, and management had begun. Whether even more rapid intervention—say, during the first couple of days—would have made a difference is doubtful, but a delay of weeks or months definitely would have made treatment more difficult.

FOUR

The Therapeutic Relationship

The first step in the use of any psychological treatment is the development of trust and collaboration. Without this, therapy is simply not possible. It is therefore of primary importance and essentially overrides any other consideration. If assessment or interventions are interfering with engagement, as opposed to facilitating it, there has to be a reconsideration of the way assessment is proceeding or how interventions are being used. Often a brief period of relaxed conversation about nonclinical issues or a pause in the therapeutic session is needed to retain and enhance engagement. However, although engagement may seem a major obstacle with many people with schizophrenia, especially where paranoia is prominent, it is not as difficult as it might at first appear.

> John had a history of paranoid schizophrenia with abuse of amphetamines and was very distrustful of authority and mental health services. He presented to the therapist who was taking over his psychiatric care with a list of demands and complaints about the response of services to his needs. By working through these individually and developing a collaborative approach to medication management, in particular, a therapeutic relationship gradually developed.

As illustrated above, engagement necessitates a certain therapeutic style that particularly emphasizes collaboration, warmth, and mutual respect. From the perspective of the person who might be distressed by accusatory auditory hallucinations, experiences of thought insertion, or persecutory fears, it takes time to begin to trust any form of therapeutic interaction.

THERAPIST ISSUES

There are a number of issues that deserve consideration when you begin to use cognitive therapy with people with schizophrenia. If you are quite new to work in mental health generally and especially with this group—and even if you are well acquainted with them—there may be a number of preconceptions that you have which are worth considering:

- How do you view people with schizophrenia?
- How do you view cognitive therapy?
- How do you view the use of cognitive therapy with people with schizophrenia?

Schizophrenia is a frightening illness to many people—including some clinicians—associated disproportionately with images of aggression, inaccessibility, and unremitting deterioration. This is strongly reinforced by the mass media, and so, unless you've been completely removed from it, it is likely to have influenced you. Schizophrenia is also associated frequently with an exclusively biological cause accompanied by the implicit assumption that only a biological solution is likely to be effective. As we discussed previously, there are certainly biological factors relevant to vulnerability and also psychosocial ones. But just as, for example, physiotherapy—a nonbiological treatment—can help people with strokes (or cardiovascular accidents), which are obviously biological, evidence also suggests that psychological therapy can help people with schizophrenia (see Chapter 2).

What other concerns might you have? Commonly people express fears, derived in part from early psychoanalytic teaching, that, first, it is not possible to form a relationship with people with schizophrenia—as Freud himself contended. Second, therapists may believe that the patient's psychosis may effectively engulf anyone trying to work psychologically with him or her. A brief review of the evidence and case studies that we have presented should, we hope, be sufficient to dispel the former fear. As to the latter, we have been working with many psychologists, nurses, and psychiatrists, and we have no reason to believe that the patient's psychosis effectively engulfs the therapist. It is, however, just such issues that need to be discussed with an experienced supervisor, if available, or with one's peers.

Working with people with schizophrenia using cognitive therapy has been for us and many others a very exciting and enriching experience. However, because so many of the techniques used seem such good "common sense," some of our trainees have felt quite deskilled and frustrated with themselves—that they have not used these techniques before (see examples in Kingdon & Turkington, 2002). As time passes, the positive aspects of working this way—and the skill involved in working with complex problems—tend to counter this initial sense of frustration.

ENGAGEMENT

Engagement with therapy varies from person to person, and some of the factors that enhance and impair it are listed in Table 4.1. Taking account of these factors can assist in determining the tactics to use in engagement.

Table 4.2 describes techniques that can assist in the engagement process. It is certainly important that communication be, as far as possible, between equals, with respect accorded to beliefs—however seemingly bizarre or irrational. It may be difficult to accept that such beliefs have meaning, but it is rare for them not be comprehensible—and if you don't understand them, don't give up. With sufficient persistence on your part, and assistance from your client, you will eventually understand them.

Befriending has proved a remarkably interesting intervention and valuable in maintaining engagement with people. It simply means being a friend to the person (as far as that is possible in a professional relationship)—for example, behaving in a similar way to how you would if visiting a work colleague in the hospital or making a visit to welcome a

TABLE 4.1. **Engagement**

Who might present particular difficulties? Someone who . . .
- Is from a different culture
- Is a substance misuser
- Has a personality disorder
- Has paranoia
- Is hostile
- Is grandiose ("Why should I?")
- Is noncompliant
- Does not see the need for help
- Believes that expressing feelings is "wrong"
- Believes that accepting help equals weakness
- Experiences negative attitudes from family and friends
- Lacks insight, with strong delusional conviction
- Is alienated from services (e.g., involuntarily detained in the hospital, has had bad experiences with hospitalization or staff, or with unpleasant drug side effects, seclusion, or restraint)
- Feels "drugged up"
- Is withdrawn

Who would be more likely to engage? A person with . . .
- Borderline personality disorder (although he or she may as easily disengage)
- Abusive hallucinations (because often nothing else is helping)
- A strong wish to get out of the hospital, especially if detained there against his or her will
- A good current and past relationship with services

TABLE 4.2. **How Would You Engage a Person with Psychosis in Cognitive-Behavioral Therapy?**

Use appropriate language.
- Avoid jargon
- Find common language
- Use vocabulary suitable to the person's educational level
- Develop the use of technical language as appropriate as it can improve "distancing"—for example, one of our clients talks of "a touch of the schizophrenias," another "somatic hallucinations"

Check out your and their level of understanding with the person.

Give simple explanations of what you want to do or learn and why.
- Provide rationale

Use appropriate structure and instill hope.

Establish common goals.
- To provide "help" generally and more specifically with, for example, voices
- To develop shared understanding
- To arrange discharge from the hospital, if desired
- To reduce medication, in collaboration with the prescriber
- To advocate for the client

Let the client leave the session . . .
- With "something"for example, a new way of looking at a situation or symptom, or just a smile on his or her face
- Feeling "befriended"

TABLE 4.3. Befriending

- Focusing on neutral nonthreatening topics
- No active formulation
- No active techniques taught or used
- Nonconfrontational
- Noncolluding
- Empathic
- Supportive
- Accepting

new neighbor. It was used as "control" treatment in our initial studies but soon demonstrated that it could be an intervention that seemed effective in its own right (see Table 4.3).

Befriending was originally developed from a program run by a voluntary organization that provided social contact to people with mental health problems (Kingdon et al., 1989). As an intervention, it provided human contact with a focus on discussing neutral but engaging topics such as holidays, the weather, sports, or TV. It has proved of value, particularly when disengagement appears to be occurring—something said or assumed by the person has upset the relationship—or distressing events have been broached and have led to an increase in agitation. Shifting into conversational chat can often retrieve a situation and relationship, allowing one to return to explore significant issues at a later stage. There is no evidence that befriending alone has an enduring effect, but as an adjunct to cognitive therapy it can be invaluable.

Cognitive therapy does need to be adapted for use in schizophrenia, and this is particularly the case in relation to engagement. Beck and Young's (Young & Beck, 1980) cognitive therapy scale (see Table 4.4) is invaluable in assessing the fidelity of cognitive therapy practices and is also useful in schizophrenia with some changes in emphasis. For example, agenda setting may need to be much more flexible than in its use with depression and anxiety. Asking a person with psychosis to construct an agenda may be too difficult if distracted by voices or cognitively impaired. It may be that agendas will be implicit and develop as sessions progress. It is important that the therapist have an agenda in mind with which to negotiate but that such a negotiation be gentle and incremental. Very often during the early sessions the client will not tolerate much structure; in fact, the agenda may well be driven almost entirely by the client.

TABLE 4.4. Cognitive Therapy Scale

General therapeutic skills
- Agenda setting
- Feedback
- Understanding
- Interpersonal effectiveness
- Collaboration
- Pacing and efficient use of time

Conceptualization, strategy, and techniques
- Guided discovery
- Focusing on key cognitions and behaviors
- Strategy for change
- Application of cognitive-behavioral techniques
- Homework

Often, such complete control of the early sessions by the client is difficult for the traditional cognitive therapist—who may be eager to unveil cognitive models to socialize, formulate, or begin to manage symptoms—to accept readily. The therapist will need to display an openness to discuss a wide range of concepts and philosophies (everything from Kundaleni to existentialism and from witchcraft to astrophysics) and display an interest in any such material produced by the client. Even though this may seem to be part of the psychotic symptomatology, exploring it fully may be the best way of explaining and understanding the odd feelings and thoughts that the person is experiencing. The key principle is to work with the person's model first as joint investigators involved in a voyage of guided discovery. The confrontational therapist will have little success in developing a joint formulation.

The therapist's style with the person with psychosis should aim to include the following elements common to working with any client: empathy, genuineness, openness, and unconditional positive regard as well as respect for the person and his or her symptoms (see Table 4.5). Warmth and humor are also often helpful, allowing sessions to be enjoyable for both parties and making difficult issues easier to discuss and action points more memorable. Humor also can allow the person to stand back from symptoms and occasionally let them go without losing face. It needs to be used carefully, especially if someone is oversensitive or paranoid. If humor could be easily misconstrued as laughing at, rather than with, the individual client, it is better avoided. Be sensitive to cues from the client in this regard.

Brief pertinent reading material can be used to back up the sessions themselves. A series of leaflets has been produced for the early phase of therapy that identifies key issues surrounding the understanding of psychotic experiences (see Appendix 4). The therapist should in turn be prepared to undertake tasks set by the prospective client—for example, to read a personal poem, to go to the library, or to use the Internet to find out about, say, Buddhist views on psychotic symptoms or reports of claimed alien abductions. When the therapist undertakes to do homework on the person's model of experience, that commitment demonstrates the scientific method of hypothesis generation and testing that is an important contribution to progress.

THE IMPORTANCE OF PACING

The pace of therapy and change may also need to be considered carefully. Cognitive therapy of schizophrenia can be a slow process. It may be appropriate to set just one target for each session, with the cognitive work being followed by one pertinent and achievable piece of work to be done between sessions. When the therapy is slowly

TABLE 4.5. **Nonspecific Therapeutic Factors**

- Accurate empathy
- Nonpossessive warmth
- Unconditional positive regard
- Nonjudgmental attitude
- Genuineness
- "Word-perfect" honesty (accurate use of language; avoiding reassurance)
- Trustworthiness

TABLE 4.6. **Engagement Principles**

- Obtain sufficient information from the referral source and clinical records prior to assessment.
- Don't jump to conclusions; take comments at face value, and examine everything fully with the client.
- Persist, but retreat if distress increases.
- Use a conversational style rather than staccato questioning.
- Don't try to do too much, but keep the flow of discussion going.
- Aim for the sessions to be positive, even enjoyable, experiences as far as its reasonable to do so.

paced, paradoxically the person often makes steady, sometimes even rapid, progress. Key points in the session are made and agreed upon, with plenty of feedback and use of a "capsule summary" (succinct description of areas covered and conclusions reached) at the end. When the person is hesitant, rephrasing questions may help, but the key thing is to allow sufficient time for the person to process the question and give a reply. Often responses are affected by distractions originating in the psychotic symptoms and other causes of cognitive deficit. The client may be experiencing voices or dwelling on paranoid beliefs—for example, if the client fears the police are outside waiting to make an arrest, he or she may understandably be slow to answer your questions. On the other hand, silence can be anxiety-provoking, and long periods of silence are better avoided; keeping the flow of conversation going in a relaxed fashion is generally most effective at building a relationship (see Tables 4.6 and 4.7). A white board, flip chart, or a piece of paper to illustrate ideas and relationships may be useful. Therapy should not be or feel like a rushed process if it is to be effective.

A NONCONFRONTATIONAL APPROACH

Interactions between staff members of mental health services and people with psychosis can easily become confrontational, or the staff can end up acting in a colluding or patronizing way. Unfortunately such interactions lead to increasing isolation of the person and to symptom maintenance. Clients stop reporting their symptoms to staff members when this happens. This reduces the possibility of developing joint reality testing.

TABLE 4.7. **Techniques to Enhance Engagement**

- "Word-perfect" honesty
- "Befriending," social conversation and relevant self-disclosure
- Taking beliefs at face value
- Enhanced listening skills
- Restricting use of silence
- Managing setting in which person is seen:
    —Go for a walk, stroll around the ward with the person
    —Go to bed space rather than formal interview room
    —Get the person a cup of tea, coffee, etc.
- Use of language: avoid jargon but don't talk down to the person

Direct confrontation is still commonly seen, and this usually leads to increased conviction in the validity of the delusion. Noncollusion is important. While the therapist is trying to work on the person's explanation of what might be going on in relation to the psychotic experience, it is vital not to collude that this is in fact accepted as the explanation. Collusion will always make delusions more entrenched.

> GEORGE: I should never have lost the Battle of Waterloo and with it the Empire of France.
>
> THERAPIST: Once we get you away from captivity we can take on the British Army again, and this time we will win.

This verbal exchange is a blatant example of collusion, but less obvious collusions can repeatedly happen during the course of therapy, including, for example, leaving open the possibility that the client's model may be true—uncritically. A proper reply can best be phrased along the lines of "If this does turn out to be true, then how would it work, how much would it cost and what would the implications be?" Alternatives can be listed, with a percentage of belief attributed to each alternative. Detecting and avoiding excessive confrontation and collusion is one of the key requirements of effective supervision. Tracing the narrow path between confrontation and collusion is best done through the use of nonjudgmental questioning and guided discovery on the basis of collaborative empiricism. A person with psychosis can start to make real progress when this approach is taken by the therapist. The alternative to the foregoing interaction could therefore be:

> GEORGE: I should never have lost the Battle of Waterloo and with it the Empire of France.
>
> THERAPIST: That's interesting. Can you tell me a bit more about how you believe you got involved in this?

This is nonconfrontational, noncolluding, and shows appropriate interest. It lets the person tell you more about something that seems important to him or her and that certainly needs further exploration.

THE IMPORTANCE OF "WORD-PERFECT" ACCURACY AND CONSISTENCY

The person with psychosis may not have been used to being given sufficient time to voice his or her ideas and concerns and, when given the opportunity to do so, is often very interested in the therapist's attitudes and opinions and the way he or she expresses them.

> IAN: The Mafia has my house under surveillance.
>
> THERAPIST 1: You are certainly distressed—there must be something going on. [accurate but a bit collusive]

Or

> THERAPIST 2: Come on now, you know there is no Mafia out there. [confrontational]

Or

> THERAPIST 3: You could be right. How can we find out? [accurate but collusive]

Or

> THERAPIST 4: Tell me more about this and how we can find out more about what is
> happening. [accurate and consistent]

Therapist 4 is likely to be the most therapeutic (accurate and consistent) in the interaction, as he or she can then move from this position to systematically work on a number of explanatory models. Similarly, if the therapist has been confrontational in prior sessions, then the person will not appreciate the switch to another style in an attempt to initiate reality testing. Therapy consistency is therefore important. If the therapist does realize that he or she has been inconsistent, then this should be openly acknowledged and the therapist can ask the person if he or she can talk about this subject from the start again. Example: "You know how I said last time that it cannot be the Mafia. Well, I think I should be a bit more open-minded. I think we should consider all the possible options." Being so accurate may seem pedantic but can make a significant difference, even when it may seem that confirming a belief is going to reinforce delusional ideas. For example, just as you are discussing paranoid beliefs, a police car siren is briefly heard. If asked, "Did you hear that?" denying or even minimizing it would simply increase suspicion. However, the implications and assumptions made can be discussed, as is also the case in this second example. The person might be discussing his or her certainty that war is breaking out—a not wholly unrealistic assessment, given the mass media's, 24/7 preoccupation with the conflicts in Iraq, the Middle East, and other locations.

THE IMPORTANCE OF COPING
WITH "INCOMPREHENSIBILITY"

Perhaps the main reason in the past for a lack of progress in psychological treatment with psychotic symptoms has been the apparent incomprehensibility of the person's symptoms. In early sessions trust is developed in the expectation that the symptoms will make sense in due course (see Table 4.8). In the same way that anxiety, depression, and phobias are psychologically understandable in terms of their formulation and content, so too are the various symptoms of schizophrenia. Any therapist new to this way of working may have difficulty believing that, but repeated experiences working with people with psychosis usually convince them. If the therapist and client can adjust to each other during the early sessions, then increased comprehensibility will start to develop as they settle down into therapy and begin to explore the prepsychotic period. This occurs after a few sessions and usually leads on to the development of a fuller case formulation (see Table 4.9).

TABLE 4.8. Commencing the Relationship

- Initially be nondirective but not aimless.
- Think about where to sit, posture, clothing, and so forth.
- Vary your interaction with the person's response (see Table 4.9):
  —Silent or monosyllabic answering
  —Interactive or overtalkative
  —Intermittent or consistent responses
  —Interruptible or noninterruptible

TACTICAL WITHDRAWAL

If there is a sudden or gradual increase in agitation or distress accompanying any particular line of questioning or investigation, it is advisable to move away from that subject matter and return to it later. Normally, talking about less distressing areas or "befriending" topics can reduce the tension so that the interview can be terminated amicably.

When differences emerge and the person becomes confrontational to the therapist—"You don't believe me, do you?"—"agreeing to differ" is a nonconfrontational way out that temporarily bypasses the subject matter and/or enables a different approach to be taken. For example:

TABLE 4.9. Coping with Different Responses

If silent:
- Have patience.
- Allow for "cognitive impairment."
- Allow for distraction and poor concentration.
- Introduce yourself and give the reason for the interview.
- Repeat greeting or simple questions (e.g., "How are you?").
- Rephrase (e.g., "Do you mind me sitting here and chatting a bit?").

If still no response:
- "Is this a bad day? Do you want me to come back some other time?"
- Just sit next to the person for a few minutes and then say goodbye and return a day or two later.
- If any nonverbal response is elicited, try relevant chat for a while (e.g., about TV if the person is watching it, or anything happening in the environment).

If answering is monosyllabic:
- Choose engaging topics.
- Use prior knowledge and the ward nurse's assistance.
- Discuss TV if watching it, ward events, weather, family, and the like.
- Self-disclosure: describe who you are and why you are speaking to the person.
- "Befriend," chat informally.
- Focus on areas responded to.

If overtalkative:
- Interruptible: let flow, and then start to interject questions when possible.
- Noninterruptible:
  —Listen.
  —Interrupt during a pause for breath or use hands to signal "hold on!"
  —Use deep pronounced breaths to signal "phew" or "wait for me"—use humor.

"I can see how important this is to you, and we don't seem to be able to agree about exactly what this all means. Perhaps we can agree to differ and leave this topic for the moment and talk about other things" [ideally mention something specific of interest to the person to discuss].

WORKING WITH DIFFERENT GROUPS

The nature of cognitive therapy is that it seeks out people's beliefs in a collaborative and nonjudgmental way, and so it can be expected to overcome issues of gender, race, age, and background. However, we may be making serious errors in assuming all this. Recently we looked at data from a large effectiveness study of cognitive therapy in schizophrenia and analyzed it by the participants' cultural background. Initially we had found that it was difficult to recruit non-Caucasian participants, but nevertheless we did recruit over 10% of the sample from these groups. But we then found that they were more likely to drop out of the study (and increased insight led, paradoxically, to increased dropout rates), and when such participants remained in the study, they were less likely to improve in terms of symptoms and insight. While the study included one black therapist, from South Africa, most non-Caucasian participants were from the Caribbean. Thus, while many cognitive therapy studies have been multicultural we need to take more measures to make them more representational and valid across cultures.

Therapist–client engagement may be particularly problematic across cultures, and style, process, and content may all be relevant. Discussions with black cognitive therapists generally reveal that their style differs in language, tone, and emphases from that of nonblack therapists—as do the symptoms. The ideal, therefore, may be to have a therapist from the person's own culture—but that may restrict members of some cultures significantly from receiving appropriate levels of therapy because of the limited availability of trained and experienced therapists. It may be that *supervision* by a therapist from the person's background could help. Perhaps the most practical way of handling this difficult issue is to accept that some cross-cultural therapy is inevitable for now, but that this needs to be discussed explicitly and opportunities provided for the person to have a therapist from their own background whenever possible.

Gender is a similar issue, and it is important not to automatically assume that cognitive therapy by its nature can overcome gender issues. Some men and some women can talk with and trust people of the same or opposite gender more easily. This will particularly be the case where sexual issues are central to therapy—or where issues relating to current male or female roles in society are relevant. Again, it seems best to allow free choice whenever possible—and especially reassess this course if progress is not made or people drop out of therapy.

Finally, a variety of other groups have specific issues that should be taken into account. People who misuse substances or have personality disorders are examples, and further discussion of these issues occurs later (in Chapter 12). Paranoia can also be expected to interfere—where this is prominent, it is generally advisable to focus on befriending and other ways of developing the therapeutic relationship before much therapy work, even assessment and formulation, is done (see Table 4.10).

TABLE 4.10. **Engaging with Different Groups**

- Defined as those from a different culture, gender, age, or background from yourself.
- General principle—match cultures, etc.—but this may exclude minority groups in practice.
- Perhaps use supervision arrangements to find therapist from the same culture.
- Reconsider if person fails to progress or drops out of therapy.
- Substance misusers: especially avoid being judgmental.
- People with personality disorder: work on empathizing through understanding life circumstances.
- Paranoia: "befriending" seems to help.
- Consider:
  —Style
  —Acknowledge differences
  —Adapt but do not imitate
  —Elicit basic assumptions about services, therapy, research, etc.
  —Alternative explanations: consider cultural/spiritual difference
    o African Caribbean, African American
    o Native American
    o African
    o Asian

TAPING SESSIONS

If the person is agreeable to sessions being audiotaped, he or she can often gain a great deal from replaying these tapes of sessions on a daily basis between sessions. This applies to people with psychosis who are suffering from not only positive but also negative symptoms and especially cognitive symptoms of impaired attention and recall. Much of this early homework can be "osmotic," enabling questioning techniques to gradually be used and rational views to emerge. The fact that the audiotape is given to the person usually limits incorporation of the therapy sessions within paranoid delusional systems. However, with the very paranoid person it is better not to attempt to introduce audiotaping until later in therapy, as suggesting taping—with its heavy association with police or secret service surveillance—may increase any existing suspicions about the therapy and therapist. The tapes are of course invaluable for supervision purposes with the person's consent. Videotaping at least occasional sessions is even more valuable in supervision, as here the body language of the client and the therapist and the extent of collaboration can be more effectively judged.

SUMMARY

Building a therapeutic relationship to enable engagement is the central process in therapy. While much may be intuitive, a full understanding of the factors involved can allow even the most difficult, paranoid, thought-disordered, or catatonic person to become a participant in a process that can have a profound effect on their distress and disability.

THERAPEUTIC RELATIONSHIP

Gordon (*sensitivity psychosis*): Developing a relationship with Gordon was reasonably straightforward—on the surface. He was open to discussion, but after an initial period became more difficult to engage and started to miss sessions. An increasing focus on ways of dealing with negative symptoms and the normalization of positive symptoms seemed helpful in reestablishing and subsequently sustaining a productive collaborative way of working.

Craig (*drug-related psychosis*): The relationship has been stormy with services and careers wherever Craig has lived. However a direct frank warm approach focusing on the issues that concern him—especially the flashbacks—along with discussing his interest in music has helped. Relatively short conversational sessions, terminated when he has begun to look agitated, have kept him in therapy. A nonjudgmental approach to his drug misuse may also have helped.

Gillian (*traumatic psychosis*): Consideration has needed to be given to gender issues, although Gillian herself has seemed not to discriminate between male or female workers. Dependency has formed quickly and has been assumed to be a necessary part of establishing a relationship but one that with time will receive attention, with gradual working toward increased independence—sufficient to allow others (e.g., housing workers) to take over necessary support.

Paul (*anxiety psychosis*): Engagement was difficult initially because of Paul's suspicion of others, but as assessment progressed he relaxed and became more trusting such that he began to discuss sensitive concerns—for example, his fear of turning into a woman. However, after this session, it proved difficult to reengage him for a period, although reengagement occurred in the end—possibly the pace of work had been too fast.

FIVE

Assessment

Assessing needs, wishes, concerns, and experiences in collaboration with a person is the only way to develop a model from which to understand his or her life and the issues he or she faces. As vulnerabilities are found, strengths identified, and stressors isolated, a formulation can be developed. This formulation can then be used to select and inform the interventions relevant for that person at that time. And, of course, the assessment process itself may be cathartic and therapeutic. A baseline against which to measure change is also established. The written assessment will form an essential part of this, but there are also measures available that may provide quantification.

So, assessment is to:

- Understand the person's background, present circumstances, and concerns.
- Develop a formulation based on a stress–vulnerability model.
- Inform selection of interventions.
- Establish a baseline against which to measure change.

GENERAL PRINCIPLES

Assessment never ends until therapy itself finishes. Even as the final discussion leading to termination of therapy occurs, information may be provided that can affect risk assessment or information that is relevant and useful to the person him- or herself and for those who will continue to be involved with him or her. On rare occasions termination itself may be reconsidered. Before that, each session will build on the initial information received before and during the very first interview.

REFERRAL INFORMATION

Information provided before initial face-to-face assessment may come in the form of written or verbal communication and be very variable in quality and comprehensiveness. It has the potential to seriously distort or significantly inform that first contact. It certainly needs to be comprehensive enough to know whether there are areas where there is any risk to the person him- or herself or to the therapist in that first interview. This should involve any incidents where the person has seriously harmed him- or herself or been aggressive to others and provide relevant details. Previous records may be available, and reading these may be illuminating. Discussion with mental health workers and significant others who know the person can be very useful in knowing the issues that may make engagement difficult or areas that the person may have difficulties discussing. However, in the absence of information or where no incidents are described, it is still appropriate to tread cautiously. Whenever the person is becoming agitated or irritable, assessment may need to be redirected or terminated.

COMMENCING ASSESSMENT

Assessment is rarely, if ever, a tidy sequential process that can be completed and then therapy start. Assessment builds and shifts focus, exploring more sensitive areas as the person is able to handle them without becoming unduly distressed. As trust builds, so the person will say more, insensitive exploration of painful areas may lead to the person's closing up—even totally disengaging and refusing to continue. It may also be the case that assessment cannot continue until some positive therapeutic benefit is achieved. This may be an improved understanding of their symptoms and situation or some specific way of coping that is developed or encouraged. Subsequently, areas of difficulty may be opened to discussion. Engagement and assessment go hand in hand, and all the considerations discussed in the preceding chapter apply.

Assessment is therefore a matter of timing and sensitivity as well as information gathering. It involves feedback at regular intervals in a manner that clarifies and consolidates but does not simply seem repetitive. An irritated "Yes, I just said that" from the client can be a response to pedantic and uninspired feedback, in contrast to "Yes, that's right."

Initially general open-ended questions can allow:

- The person's primary concerns to be voiced.
- A focus on the person rather than the therapist.
- The process of engagement to develop.
- Useful information to be obtained.

A brief introduction might involve asking, "How are you feeling today?" but needs to be responsive to the person's demeanor, previous information, and whatever he or she said on first meeting the therapist. If the person looks very depressed or agitated or confused, it may be reasonable to say that he or she is looking "down" or "low" and make further assessment of the responses. Correctly identifying the person's mood empathically may quickly build a therapeutic alliance. If in doubt, however, a more general question is safer, for example, "How long have things not been so good?"

It may be better to avoid any mention of illness—for example, asking "How long have you been ill?"—until you are clear that this terminology is acceptable. He or she may respond to such a question with "I'm not ill," and such an exchange can impair engagement.

Responding to the individual's statements involves commenting on that person's perception of his or her mood—"I'm sorry you feel like that" or "Can you tell me what's been making you feel that way?" He or she may give a neutral or guarded response such as "I'm OK" or "I'm fine." When people with schizophrenia seem—or you've been told that they are—suspicious of people generally and mental health staff in particular, a very general follow-up question ("Can you tell me about what's been happening to you?") rather than a more specific one ("What sorts of problems have you been having?") may be the better way to proceed.

Assessment of his or her problems may then involve a process of gentle exploration. Questioning can be quite direct, if sensitive and gentle. "What?" "Why?" and "How?" can assist in elucidating issues effectively. But there is a point at which broadening the assessment to explore background information becomes necessary. In general, this is probably best done once the initial presenting problem has been clarified—but probably before its history is explored in much detail. However, it should be only when the person is ready to change directions. If the person wishes to explore a specific issue further and is even mildly distressed or irritated by an attempted shift to other areas, it is best to continue on the current subject matter until that line of inquiry is exhausted.

FULL ASSESSMENT

A fully comprehensive assessment involves understanding the personal, social, medical, and mental health history as well as the presenting problem or symptoms. However, circumstances may dictate that assessment is truncated, or as experience is gained, it may be possible to focus on specific areas. For example, on first presentation, little information may be available and the person may be uncooperative. Assessment still needs to be as full as possible, but there may be severe limitations put upon it. Often it is assumed that exploring early development of beliefs or personal history will be difficult in such circumstances, but this is not necessarily so, and it is generally worth trying to gauge response to discussion of these areas. Paradoxically, temporarily taking the emphasis off the current concerns that led to the distress and conflict can sometimes improve the relationship such that returning later to deal with current issues becomes easier. Rather than have the therapist seen as just interested in problems, a more holistic approach can be attractive to people with schizophrenia. However, if a person says that he or she does not want to talk about something, it is essential that that be respected—the person will return to it when he or she feels able to. Even if the person just seems uneasy, it is essential that he or she be offered the opportunity to stop: "Is this discussion upsetting you at all? We can stop or talk about something else if you like?" Even if the person says he or she wishes to continue, it can be worth checking: "Are you sure?"

Assessing Personal History

Once the initial problems have been described, these can be detailed and refined. The history of how they developed can be explored, or you can change tack altogether and ask about the personal history. While it might seem to be bringing in irrelevant material and losing the direction of the interview, it is very frequently a way of providing structure and understanding. As the person develops his or her story, so the way in which beliefs have developed is put into context. A logical progression develops from understanding vulnerabilities and strengths to assessment of relevant stressful circumstances and then the impact of distress and disability.

> "Thanks. That clarifies the problems, and I do want to discuss that in more detail. But it would help if we can put that in context, just get an understanding of how this developed. That may mean that some of the questions I ask may seem a bit unrelated to your current situation, but it helps us get an understanding of the broad picture. Is that OK?
>
> "So, . . . did you grow up around here? . . . Where were you born?"

Table 5.1 gives an outline of the areas needing to be covered. Essentially this is a generic mental health assessment—the table is not intended to be comprehensive but to set out key areas. It is included to ensure that these areas are not omitted and also because considerable variation exists among practitioners and services in what is considered a comprehensive assessment. In practice, after establishing key reasons for referral, as previously mentioned it is often easier and clearer to elicit all other areas of the assessment before returning to the history of the development of the key problems. This is because complex histories of current circumstances often introduce elements from the history of mental health problems and personal history in a way that is clarified by earlier systematic exploration.

It may be that—for a 75-year-old—issues about childhood seem a bit distant, and it is certainly important to weigh the benefits of asking these questions against the possible irritation they may cause. However, so often, vitally important information emerges that has direct relevance to current concerns. Simply because the focus will be

---

TABLE 5.1. Assessment Areas

- Referral method (i.e., emergency, routine, referral source)
- Reasons for referral (from person him- or herself, caregivers, and referring agent)
  —History of the development of these reasons
- Personal history
  —Birth
  —Early development
  —Schooling
  —Work history
  —Relationships: friends, sexual partners
- Family history (especially current situation and relationships)
  —Parents, brothers, and sisters (relevant others)
  —Partner, children (if any)
  —Any family experience of mental health problems
- Social circumstances (especially accommodation and finances)
- Substance use (alcohol and illicit drugs)
- Forensic history (contacts with police and courts)
- Physical health (including past and current serious illnesses or accidents)
- Mental health history, past contacts with mental health care systems

---

on the "here-and-now"—specifically, cognitions, behavior, and emotion—does not mean that how the person got to the "here-and-now" can be ignored. Relationships with others are particularly important, as frequently relevant issues to psychotic symptoms emerge.

The questioning may become rather one-sided, but often people will get into the flow of describing their lives and then simply need prompting and to be asked for occasional clarification. From all this, a vulnerability-stress model can quite rapidly emerge. For many people this will be the first time they have ever been through such a description of their lives, at least since their first contact with mental health services, and as well as enabling assessment this can be a significant therapeutic process.

Assessing Time and Circumstances of Onset

Establishing the initial point when problems began to develop is necessary to understand continuing symptoms. The sequential life history assists with this, but the specific point or period of onset may be missed and may require direct inquiry:

- "When were you first unwell?"
- "When did things first start going wrong for you?"
- "When did you first go to see a psychiatrist or psychologist?"

Assessing and understanding the antecedents—preceding events and circumstances—leading up to the onset of psychotic symptoms themselves is crucial to later therapeutic work. Understanding what the person was doing, feeling, or thinking prior to developing the problems can allow both the therapist and the client to see why he or she came to the conclusions he or she did or experienced the symptoms that emerged. It may be necessary to use a range of sources including:

- Report from the individual him- or herself
- Families
- Friends
- Neighbors
- Staff members who have known him or her previously
- Previous psychiatric records
- Records from other sources (where available and accessible and, generally, with the person's permission)
- Family doctors or general practitioners
- Other medical notes
- Social workers
- Criminal records
- Local newspapers where circumstances of specific reported events are relevant

Through these routes a picture of the buildup to the development of symptoms can be constructed and related to the symptoms themselves. The relevant events and circumstances will very frequently relate directly to the content of the current beliefs or hallucinations.

Julie had been brought up in a series of foster homes after her mother abandoned her as a young child. From the age of 7 to 10, she was sexually abused by one of her foster fathers. This occurred at a regular time during the day, lunchtime, when her foster mother was out doing part-time work. In the room where the abuse occurred, the television was always on. In later life, she would get visual hallucinations reflecting the content of the TV programs that were on at that time, accompanied by her foster father's voice threatening her and telling her that she was evil.

Taking the psychiatric history can give the therapist an understanding of how beliefs developed, often complicated by the secondary effects of hospitalization, medication, and stigmatization, which may confuse or reinforce beliefs, especially paranoid ones (e.g., the procedures attending admission to a hospital can often reinforce paranoid beliefs by being seen as unreasonable by the person involved and confirming existing beliefs).

Understanding Motivating Factors and Life Goals

Understanding motivating factors may occur spontaneously but, equally, may not. Ask the person: "What do you like doing?" or "What would you like to do in the future—say in 5 years time?" If he or she does not know, prompting is reasonable to do: "What about an occupation or relationships with other people—that is, having a girl- or boyfriend and other friends, a family, a job that provides some money for you."

Assessing Symptoms

Assessing symptoms often flows out of the foregoing conversations. Nevertheless, certain symptoms may require more direct inquiry. The problems may be that asking directly about paranoia or voices may prompt the response "You think I'm mad, don't you?" and impair engagement. This is possibly an area where specific inquiry can be left to a later stage. However, it is very important to have an understanding of the variety of psychotic symptoms that exist (as described in Chapter 1) and be able to elicit which ones apply to the client. Questions used in diagnostic instruments for DSM-IV-TR and ICD-10 classification systems and rating scales for psychosis are useful to know but need to be used sensitively—simply asking a series of seemingly unrelated questions can cause a very negative reaction in clients. The symptoms are best elicited in relation to the events that have affected the person and the context immediately explored.

Hallucinations are often elicited by asking "Do you ever hear people talking when there doesn't seem to be anyone around?" or "Do you ever hear things that other people don't seem to hear?" or "Do you see things that others don't seem to see or that appear in places you wouldn't expect them?" Delusions often emerge in conversation and are so varied that specific questions can miss them. But if the person seems suspicious or distressed, commence by asking "Is there anything worrying you?" or "Are you getting on with people reasonably well?" This often provides material that can be explored further. Asking questions that seem to have no relevance to the conversation can increase suspicion "You are just trying to trap me" or "You think I'm mad, don't you?"—and impair the development of a therapeutic relationship.

General discussion often leads to specific symptoms being described, and usually enough material about symptoms will come out to make a therapeutic start. Questions about sleep ("How's your sleep?") or appetite ("Are you eating all right? Have you lost weight recently?") may provide opportunities for people to talk about worries they have, perhaps keeping them awake at night ("What sorts of things are going through your mind while you are trying to get to sleep?"). Asking about relationships, friendships ("Have you got a few friends?"), or neighbors ("Do you see much of your neighbors?") can lead into discussion of paranoid beliefs, social phobia, isolation, delusions of reference, and so forth. The initial discussion of "How are you feeling?" can lead delicately into a discussion of "Do you sometimes feel you don't want to go on anymore?"—becoming a more explicit exploration of suicidal beliefs.

Although a focus on psychotic symptoms is necessary, this can distract from comprehensive assessment and later therapy. Depression, anxiety, confusion, and anger can be at least as important for many people as voices and strong beliefs.

Assessment of Substance Use

Use of alcohol, nicotine, and illicit drugs is very common in people with mental health problems as well as the general population. Assessment of amounts consumed and their effects on the individual needs to be done in a nonjudgmental way. The reasons for consumption also need to be understood.

Alcohol

Measurement in units of alcohol ("drinks") is a useful way of gauging quantity, but effects will vary. For someone who has had long-standing problems with alcohol any alcohol may be problematic, while for others its use may be appropriate in social circumstances for relaxation and developing friendships and relationships.[1] Prohibition may simply add another difficulty to an already problematic area. So, assessment of the effect on the individual needs to be specific—"How much do you drink? How often? What effects does it have? Why do you drink that much?" Assessment for dependence may be necessary, and various tools exist for this. Inquiry into how problems began may identify alcohol as a component, or other pointers may indicate that it has become one.

Cannabis

Assessment of the effects of cannabis can be difficult but necessary. As an illegal substance (in countries where this is the case), the risks of consuming it may bring added stress, either directly from police activity or indirectly from fear of being caught, or may simply heighten financial problems and attendant symptoms. A client's associating with people regularly misusing drugs can lead to paranoid beliefs about, for example, drug dealers being out to find and harm the client. Many people with and without psychosis however describe relaxation as a prominent effect, and there may be social pressure to

---

[1]Up to two drinks per day for men and one drink per day for women and older people is not harmful for most adults. (A standard drink is one 12-ounce bottle or can of either beer or wine cooler, one 5-ounce glass of wine, or 1.5 ounces of 80-proof distilled spirits.)

participate in its use. For others, the effects of cannabis can depress, confuse, or specifically precipitate or exacerbate psychotic symptoms. Above all, assessing the variety of responses that the person has to the drug and working out what to do about them needs to be a collaborative activity taking into account all positive and negative factors.

Amphetamines, Cocaine, Ecstasy, LSD

Again, assessing the specific effect is necessary, but even social use of these drugs seems to lead to problems much more frequently in people vulnerable to psychosis.

Opiates

Again, assessment is appropriate, but in practice, at least in the United Kingdom, it is very rare for opiate abusers to receive a diagnosis of schizophrenia or for those with such a diagnosis to become dependent on, or even use, these drugs to any great extent.

Nicotine

Unfortunately, the use of nicotine, usually in cigarettes, is extremely high. Assessment of the amount, attempts to discontinue its use, and the reasons for continuing to need it should be sought out and discussed.

Forensic History

Harm to self is much more common than harm to others, and general criminal activity is no more frequent than in the general population. It seems most related to any concurrent substance misuse. However, knowledge of any forensic history may be very relevant, as frequently it coincides with onset or relapse of symptoms. Where this is not the case, it may be relevant at a later stage, as these issues may lead to difficulties in, for example, finding living accommodations and work.

Assessing Social Circumstances

An understanding of the person's current contacts, living arrangements, financial situation, and interests is essential because it can be very difficult to use cognitive therapy without appreciating the client's major concerns with social circumstances. However, it may still be possible and indeed desirable to use cognitive therapy as a way of eliciting the reasons why the person is in difficulties and finding acceptable ways out—as case manager to the person or in collaboration with the case manager. Social interaction style can affect development of relationships and also be relevant. Current friendships, family and staff, educational level, and the like are all relevant in terms of what supports and protective factors are present.

Assessing Risk

An assessment of risk to self or others is an essential part of any initial and continuing assessment. This needs to be done before assessment takes place on the basis of the available information and further information sought if any concerns arise. During assessment and as therapy proceeds, this needs to be continued and appropriate advice sought and action taken if concerns arise. Past behavior remains the most reliable predictor of future behavior. Risk to self is much more common than risk to others, and risk in psychosis is similar in frequency to that in mood disorders (lifetime suicide rates are estimated at 10–15%). Cognitive therapy practiced by trained therapists or those being effectively supervised has not been shown to increase these risks and indeed may reduce them, but caution and attention to risk factors are always needed.

Initial Formulation of the Problem List

Having completed the initial assessment, the presenting problem will usually have been articulated by the person. It may present as a symptom—"my voices"—or accusation against others—"I haven't got a problem if people would just leave me alone"—or something more specific and practical—"I don't like my flat." As the assessment proceeds, a number of possible problems may emerge and can be listed with the person: "So, you're having trouble sleeping, the neighbors are upsetting you, and you can't go out. That's certainly enough to make a start with, but is there anything else you'd like to add?"

Diagnostic Interviews

Interviews using diagnostic schedules for ICD-10 and DSM-IV-TR, mentioned previously, are available and can be useful in eliciting diagnostic features but are too unwieldy in most clinical settings. In most instances where referral is made for cognitive therapy, diagnosis will have been made previously by a psychiatrist—although, as assessment proceeds, this may need reviewing. Where there are issues of uncertainty, it may be that further evaluation of this may be appropriate.

As we have described earlier (in Chapter 1), we have found it helpful to use four clinical subgroups of the broad category of schizophrenia, and these may overlap with other diagnostic entities such as borderline personality disorder and depressive psychosis. Using a continuum diagnostic model such as that represented in Figure 5.1 can

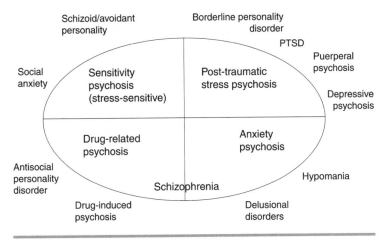

FIGURE 5.1. Clinical subgroups and related conditions.

be helpful. For example, frequently there is confusion and debate as to whether a person has a borderline personality disorder or schizophrenia—they may meet criteria for both. Therapy would involve work with both the psychotic symptoms and the issues to do with the borderline personality disorder. As the person becomes able to, for example, reattribute the voices being heard to their own thoughts, so the issues about content of those voices—often related to previous traumatic events—become accessible to work with. In effect, the work on borderline personality disorder then takes over from that on the psychotic symptoms.

Similarly, social anxiety and paranoia seem to be on a continuum possibly with sensitivity disorder, although paranoia can also be a feature of the other groups (see Chapter 13 for further discussion). It may be helpful to decide which group the individual seems most likely to belong to—if any. Management may be helpfully organized, as described later (in Chapter 6), following development of the formulation.

Rating Questionnaires

Identifying and quantifying symptoms and social circumstances by using rating scales can be very valuable in training and evaluation. However, there are dangers that their use can be a substitute for good comprehensive assessment, and they can be used in a mechanical way, interfering with engagement. When used, they need to be introduced after a relationship with the person has been established, the initial problems understood, and personal history clarified. This often means that it is not possible to use the first session for quantifying symptoms in any detail, but this needs to be done subsequently. Rating scales certainly need to be introduced carefully. They are used:

- To help you and the person him- or herself to identify key issues.
- To measure change so that progress can be identified—overall and in specific areas.
- To provide material to help with supervision and training.
- To provide information for those paying for the service or overseeing it—and where this is the case, it is important that the person be aware of this.

Use of research questionnaires in clinical practice is restricted by the time consumed in completing them. So, the Positive and Negative Syndrome Scale (PANSS), Scale for the Assessment of Negative Symptoms (SANS), Social Behavior Schedule (SBS), and Comprehensive Psychopathological Rating Scale (CPRS) have proved valuable in research studies but are not much used by clinicians. They may, however, be valuable in assessing specific symptoms and useful in training because of the definitions of symptoms that they provide.

More accessible are scales or global rating measures that are briefer (see Table 5.2). At one end is the Global Assessment of Functioning (GAF), which is simple to complete and used widely in the United States. More lengthy to complete are the Brief Psychiatric Rating Scale (BPRS) and Manchester Scales (MS), which provide more information on psychotic symptoms. In the United Kingdom, the development of the Health of the Nation Outcome Scale (HoNOS), designed for use as a reliable measure of social and psychological change, has much to commend it. Its range (see Table 5.3 and Appendix 1) includes those issues that are key targets in psychosocial interventions such as cogni-

TABLE 5.2. Rating Instruments

Applicable to most clients
- Health of the Nation Outcome Scale
- Psychotic Symptoms Rating Scales
- Global Assessment of Functioning

Applicable to some
- Beck Depression Inventory
- Scale for the Assessment of Negative Symptoms

tive-behavioral therapy, and it is simple to rate on a 0–4 scale. Reliability has been an issue, but training in its use is recommended to overcome this.

HoNOS is limited in its assessment of specific symptoms, and supplementation can be considered with individual people. Dimensional measures of psychotic symptoms can assist assessment. The Psychotic Symptoms Rating Scales (PSYRATS) do this effectively for hallucinations and delusions (see Tables 5.4 and 5.5 and Appendix 2). Use of measures to assess and manage depression may also be worth considering, for example, the Beck Depression Inventory (BDI). Beliefs about voices as measured by questionnaire (Chadwick's BAVQ) can also be worth considerating. Inventories to measure self-esteem (e.g., Noble's) and quality of life may be relevant but have not yet been shown to change in research trials, so would not be expected to demonstrate much change in clinical practice. Additional measures to assess specific problems such as insight (Birchwood or David Insight Scales), assertiveness (Rathus Assertiveness Scale), or anger (e.g., the Novaco Anger Scale) may also be worth consideration.

In summary, there are a variety of scales that can be valuable as training aids or for clinical usage (see Table 5.6). The use of a broad scale, such as HoNOS or GAF, is recommended with a scale specifically measuring psychotic symptoms, such as PSYRATS. Where negative symptoms, depression, and the like are a key focus of the intervention, scales to measure these are available and can assist assessment and measurement of change.

TABLE 5.3. Health of the Nation Outcome Scale (HoNOS)

- Overactive or aggressive behavior
- Nonaccidental self-injury
- Problem drinking or drug taking
- Cognitive problems
- Physical symptoms
- Problems associated with hallucinations or delusions
- Problems with depression
- Other symptoms—specify
- Problems with
  ... relationships
  ... daily living
  ... living conditions
  ... occupation and activities

TABLE 5.4. Psychotic Symptoms Rating Scales: Dimensions of Hallucinations

- Frequency
- Duration
- Location
- Loudness
- Beliefs about origin
- Amount of negative content of voices
- Degree of negative content of voices
- Amount of distress
- Frequency of distress
- Disruption to life
- Controllability of voices

TABLE 5.5. Psychotic Symptoms Rating Scales: Dimensions of Delusions

- Amount of preoccupation with delusions
- Duration of preoccupation with delusions
- Conviction (at time of interview)
- Amount of distress
- Frequency of distress
- Disruption to life

TABLE 5.6. Examples of Rating Scales

Scale	Authors (year)
Global Assessment of Functioning (GAF)	Endicott et al. (1976)
Brief Psychiatric Rating Scale (BPRS)	Overall & Graham (1962)
Manchester Scales (MS)	Krawiecka et al. (1977)
Health of the Nation Outcome Scale (HoNOS)	Wing et al. (1998)
Positive and Negative Syndrome Scale (PANSS)	Kay et al. (1987)
Scale for the Assessment of Negative Symptoms (SANS)	Andreasen (1981)
Social Behavior Schedule (SBS)	Birchwood et al. (1990)
Comprehensive Psychopathological Rating Scale (CPRS)	Asberg et al. (1978)
Psychotic Symptoms Rating Scale (PSYRATS)	Haddock et al. (1999)
Beck Depression Inventory (BDI)	Beck et al. (1961)
Beliefs About Voices Questionnaire (BAVQ)	Chadwick et al. (2000)
Self-Esteem Scale	Robson (1989)
Birchwood Insight Scale	Birchwood et al. (1994)
David Insight Scale	David (1990)

ASSESSMENT

Gordon *(sensitivity psychosis)*: Assessment with Gordon did not raise any difficult issues. He was fully cooperative, but useful information was given by his mother, and contact with her was of significant assistance, as family issues were clarified. Elucidating negative symptoms was one area of complexity.

Craig *(drug-related psychosis)*: Thought disorder and impulsivity interfered with assessment, as Craig's concentration span was poor and he was easily distracted, particularly in discussing any emotionally charged issues. This meant that assessment was supplemented by information from records and only slowly confirmed with him. Discussing personal history was difficult to do sequentially, but a jigsaw of key parts eventually came together. Risk assessment has been a prominent concern because of his suicidal thoughts and past actions.

Gillian *(traumatic psychosis)*: Assessment was not easy with Gillian, as the difficulties in building trust and her limited intelligence meant that engagement took priority. This meant that assessment was slow and involved drawing information from a variety of sources as well as her own statements. Understandably, the circumstances surrounding the traumatic events occurring to her were particularly sensitive and were proceeded with very gently at the pace that she was able to cope with—without causing distress sufficient to more than transiently increase her symptoms.

Paul *(anxiety psychosis)*: Assessment of background information was more straightforward—as is often the case with anxiety psychosis. Paul was able to describe the circumstances in which he had developed the beliefs that he held and some of the delusional ideas. But because of the embarrassing and disturbing nature of some, he avoided discussing these in detail. However, as the relationship developed, he was able to discuss them and able to participate in rating them—on HoNOS, risk of suicide was noted, along with depression and psychotic symptoms scores, and limited social interaction was also picked up. With PSYRATS, he scored highly on most of the scales, especially in terms of conviction, distress, and preoccupation.

SIX

Individualized Case Formulation and Treatment Planning

Case formulation develops out of the assessment process and will sometimes guide it. As your experience grows, it becomes increasingly apparent that certain features occur together, and so you will inevitably be particularly interested in eliciting them. The subgroups that we delineated in Chapter 1 emerge from such a process. However, it is very important not to prejudge people: they do not necessarily fit the patterns we weave for them. Assessment and formulation need to be an open frank exchange of views, and it is particularly important to cover all relevant areas of personal and mental health history.

A case formulation provides a framework from which to develop therapeutic interventions, and constructing it in itself can be therapeutic. Providing a way of understanding the different elements in the person's life that have combined to lead to the current problems can allow the person him- or herself with—or sometimes without—further support to address them. Usually a collaborative process of focusing on specific issues develops.

The specific formulation that you deduce can be written down on a white board or large paper sheet, but you do need to be aware of how such an approach will be viewed by the person. Some find it intimidating, particularly where:

- Schooling has been a negative experience,
- Their literacy is limited.
- They have problems with authority figures and see this as a "teaching" approach.
- Where a particularly painful episode is being reviewed.

What is included in the formulation presented to the person also needs consideration. For some people, a simple diagram linking stress to vulnerability may be sufficient (see Figure 6.1): This can be explained by demonstrating, using the diagram, that some people have a very low level of vulnerability but a level of stress so high that they become ill (A in Figure 6.1), whereas others may be very vulnerable, in which case rela-

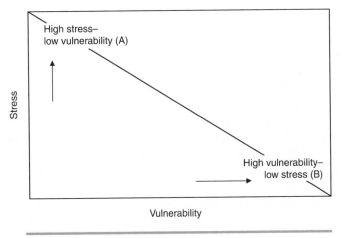

FIGURE 6.1. Stress–vulnerability.

tively low levels of stress can lead to illness (B). For some people, an awareness of the link between pressure and negative symptoms, especially motivation, may be enough to understand, at least initially.

But, whatever is presented, the therapist does need a clear balanced formulation from which to work. Understanding the person's background is the first step, including:

- *Predisposing or vulnerability factors*: those issues that may make the person more sensitive to stress and specifically to developing a psychotic illness (e.g., family history of mental health problems, especially psychosis; personality characteristics, such as tending to be very solitary ["schizoid"], sensitive, or paranoid; or brain injury, which may contribute to developing symptoms).
- *Precipitating factors*: those relevant experiences that immediately preceded the person becoming ill—a detailed discussion of the period building up to the first episode allows identification of factors that the person also identifies or agrees were relevant.
- *Perpetuating factors*: those issues that make full recovery more difficult or relapse more likely (e.g., lack of income, poor housing, poor treatment adherence, isolation, and difficult relationships).
- *Protective factors*: the strengths which can aid recovery (e.g., intelligence, relationships, interests, and aptitudes).

Next, identify current problems. Check whether the initial presenting problem (even if it occurred years before) remains a problem to be dealt with.

Next, clarify which thoughts, feelings, and behaviors predominate and are relevant to illness. Similarly, physical symptoms and social circumstances of relevance—whether or not identified as problems—need to be included in the formulation.

Finally, have any underlying concerns been identified? This is a more difficult area, and it may be that schematic beliefs, rules for living, or more simply general social or psychological factors that seem to be driving delusional beliefs and behavior (e.g., "I need a girlfriend," "My parents hate me") will be included here (see Chapter 9 on delu-sions for further discussion of this).

The formulation may then take the form of a paragraph or be set out diagrammati-cally (e.g., Appendix 5.1, "Making Sense"). It may be that some components (e.g., thoughts, feelings, and actions) will be particularly emphasized and others provided in less detail, but this will vary from person to person. Its content needs to be checked with the person with whom it has been developed, but the way in which this is done needs careful consideration. Factual matters may be clarified, connections discussed, and for some the diagram used in full, but it is important not to overwhelm the person. A copy may be given to the client, as well as perhaps a tape of the discussion describing it.

There will be times when the formulation cannot be agreed upon completely with the client, but establishing where the differences lie can be valuable. It is important not to be challenging over this, and if the person wants parts removed it will generally be best to do so—or, better, develop a compromise way of expressing the key disagree-ment(s).

TREATMENT PLANNING

Engagement and assessment are continuing processes throughout therapy that will en-sure that the person remains engaged and collaborative in the evolution of the formula-tion. Specific work on symptoms comes out of the formulation, for example, the initial issues leading to delusions or hallucinations will emerge, and discussion of these will almost inevitably ensue. There will then be exploration of them and alternative expla-nations by gathering relevant information from the person's own knowledge, that of the therapist, or sought from elsewhere (e.g., friends or libraries). Figure 6.2 illustrates the sequence of therapy in very broad terms, and further chapters will describe the components in more detail.

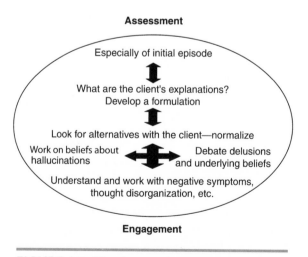

FIGURE 6.2. The therapeutic process.

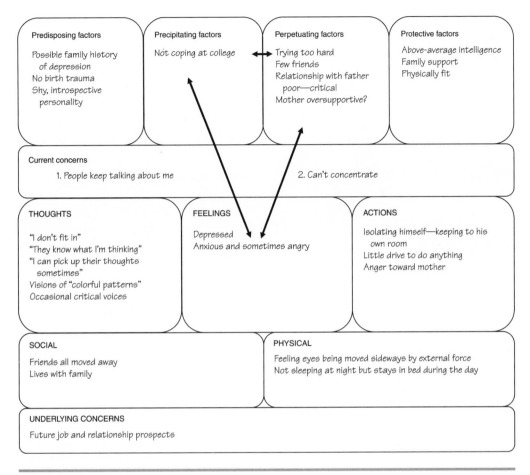

FIGURE 6.3. Gordon's *(sensitivity psychosis)* formulation.

USING THE FORMULATION

The process of developing the formulation with the client can be therapeutic in itself as a structure begins to emerge from an often disorganized group of symptoms and experiences. For Gordon and his family, as will be discussed later, a major step forward was developing an understanding of key elements, particularly the "vicious cycle" developing between deteriorating performance, "trying too hard" to compensate, and then increased anxiety and eventually demoralization, worsening performance still further (see Figure 6.3). Other factors were also relevant (e.g., isolation and poor social performance), and a treatment plan also included them.

Frequently a few linked thoughts and experiences form a key axis to work with—for example, as illustrated in the formulation in Figure 6.4, the link between flashbacks and the initial drug experience has been very important for Craig. There are other links of significance, but being able to reconceptualize the voices and control as being a "flashback" to previous drug-precipitated episodes aided his insight considerably.

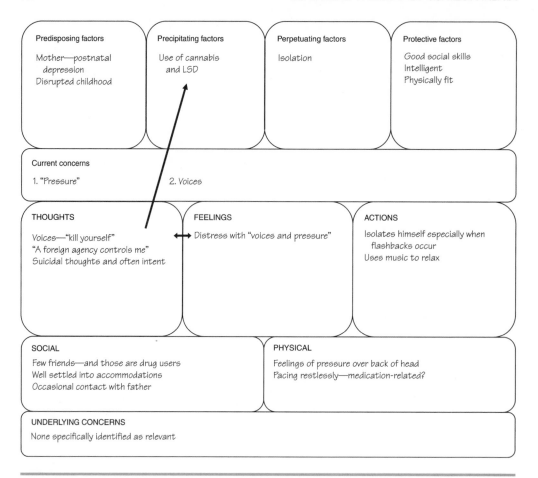

FIGURE 6.4. Craig's (*drug-related psychosis*) formulation.

Finding relevant connections can assist in reattributing symptoms—as can specific work described in later chapters on delusions and hallucinations. Strengths can be mobilized and maladaptive behaviors can be identified. However, the formulation developed with the client may need to be very simple, even though the therapist may need to build a more detailed understanding; for example, a simple diagram making the key connections was most appropriate with Gillian (see Figure 6.5).

With the client it is possible to identify and agree on key areas to work on, for example, voices, isolation, or weight loss—or all three. These can be addressed individually or (as described in later chapters) through work on underlying beliefs. This turned out to be the situation with Paul, as usually occurs with anxiety psychosis (see formulation in Figure 6.6). He was able to eventually see links between his symptoms and his situation—and possible precipitants for his illness. The conviction in his delusional beliefs persisted, but he allowed the therapist to work with him on his underlying concerns about his sexuality and his future as distinct issues.

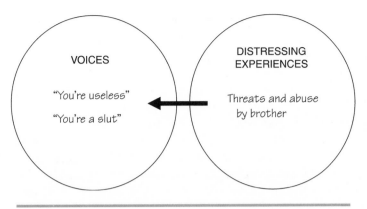

FIGURE 6.5. Gillian's *(traumatic psychosis)* formulation.

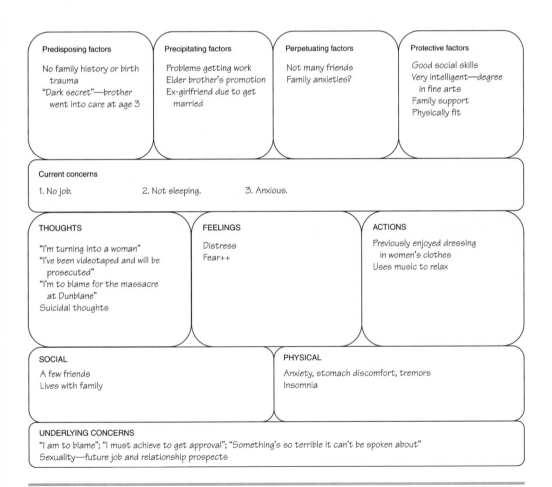

FIGURE 6.6. Paul's *(anxiety psychosis)* formulation.

SETTING TARGETS

Target setting needs to be cautious, as failure to achieve targets can affect engagement, morale, and subsequent performance. Initially the process of establishing the key concerns of the client is important, and it may then be sufficient just to convey that "what we want to do is deal with these concerns in any way we can."

As engagement is established and formulation develops, other targets may emerge—for example, "to be able to go out and cope better with other people talking about me." The therapist's goals may be "insight," but an explicit target "to stop you from believing people are talking about you" would not be collaboratively developed or appropriate at this stage for the client. Agreeing about "coping" is often a reasonable compromise position to take while not colluding in the belief.

Goals may be practical—for example, "to get a job or girlfriend"—or emotional—for example, "to reduce the distress caused by my voices." Clients may suggest targets that may be overambitious, for example, "getting rid of my voices." Negotiation can usually lead to "coping with my voices" as a more realistic goal, at least in the short term (even though some people do become free of voices over time). Setting goals for negative symptoms is discussed in detail in Chapter 12.

MANAGEMENT OF CLINICAL SUBGROUPS

Consideration of the clinical subgroups previously described can assist in identifying the type of work that is likely to be successful. It is, however, very important to ensure that it is consistent with the formulation and rooted in it. With sensitivity psychosis, negative symptoms are particularly prominent as an issue and often the prime focus of caregiver concern. Providing a clear rationale for action and sharing the formulation can overcome caregiver objections and improve collaboration with the person him- or herself. Positive symptoms frequently involve delusions of reference, thought interference, and paranoia, although a range of other disparate symptoms can present, but often with fluctuating conviction. Thought disorder can sometimes confuse communication and be exacerbated by the therapists focusing too energetically on delusional beliefs and voices (see Figure 6.7).

Work with the drug-related group involves identification and full description of the initial episodes, which enables comparison between current symptoms and earlier experiences to be made, there by facilitating reattribution. Personality factors such as schizotypal, schizoid, and antisocial traits can be prominent etiological and maintaining factors. People with schizoid and schizotypal personalities often start using drugs as part of a mystical search for meaning. Those with antisocial personalities often begin using hallucinogens as part of a personal rebellion against society. Both the search for meaning and the rebellion can be addressed within-session, with the aim of leading to a reduction in hallucinogen use. Caregivers have often been through serious crises themselves, often through relationship difficulties, and these need to be sensitively taken into account when working with clients. This is especially true where work with critical expressed emotion is an issue, as frequently it is. Collaboration over issues such as medication and activity scheduling needs a patient, negotiated, and consistent approach, which can put a strain on the therapeutic relationship from both sides (see Fig-

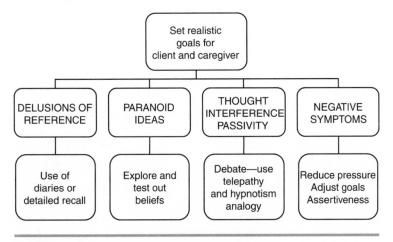

FIGURE 6.7. Management of sensitivity disorder.

ure 6.8). Continuing work on drug misuse, where needed, utilizes principles described in Chapter 13.

The dominant symptoms with traumatic psychosis, as described previously, tend to be abusive, commanding hallucinations and depressive episodes related to the past traumatic events. Work involves reattribution and work on content and underlying beliefs (see Chapter 10). Unfortunately, these voices often seem, to be resistant to medication, at least in part. Exposure work on the traumatic events themselves can be too distressing for many clients, but work on the beliefs surrounding them can be possible and successful with time (see Figure 6.9).

With anxiety psychosis (see Figure 6.10), the predominant problems tend to be the delusional beliefs, which are often systematized. Work with these is described in Chapter 9. Normalizing and developing alternative explanations are often useful, especially early on and in engagement, but techniques for dealing with resistant delusions (e.g., inference chaining and work with underlying beliefs), are usually employed to good effect.

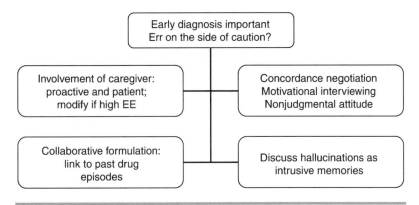

FIGURE 6.8. Management of drug-related psychosis.

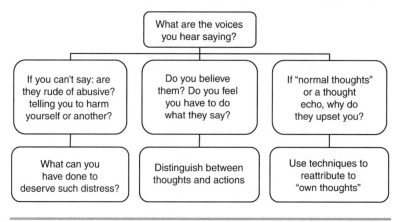

FIGURE 6.9. Management of traumatic psychosis.

INDIVIDUALIZED CASE FORMULATION AND TREATMENT

Gordon (*sensitivity psychosis*): The key issue arising from the formulation was the need to connect Gordon's stressful circumstances (i.e., school pressures and college work) to vulnerability (i.e., his quiet contemplative personality, with perpetuating factors such as the family atmosphere and expectations). A conceptualization of the problems in terms of stress sensitivity was credible to Gordon and his family. A full written formulation (Figure 6.3) was used to explain this.

Craig (*drug-related psychosis*): The essential elements involved the initial precipitant—drug misuse—and vulnerability from limited family support (Figure 6.4). The term "flashbacks" helped link the perceptions experienced to the initial episode, which was a key element in the formulation.

Gillian (*traumatic psychosis*): As assessment evolved, a simple formulation (Figure 6.5) was developed, with Gillian linking together the abusive events that had occurred and the voices she was hearing. Her vulnerabilities—associated with her limited emotional and practical skills—were included, but in a noncritical supportive way, with the emphasis on actions that could be taken to diminish them.

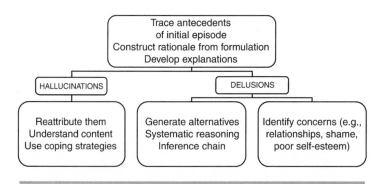

FIGURE 6.10. Management of anxiety psychosis.

Paul (*anxiety psychosis*): The importance of formulation in work with Paul can hardly be overstated (Figure 6.6). Its development was fundamentally important in allowing him to understand and appreciate the context in which his beliefs had developed. It assisted in the development of the therapeutic relationship, as the holistic approach circumvented direct confrontation over his beliefs. This enabled him to begin to examine his beliefs with the therapist. Underlying concerns about his future and sexuality played a major role in the generation and perpetuation of his symptoms which, once identified, he became prepared to work on.

SEVEN

Orienting the Client to Treatment

How explicit about cognitive therapy do you need to be? You need to strike a balance between being open and saying enough, yet not saying too much to confuse the person, especially when his or her thoughts are disordered or seriously distracted by delusional beliefs or voices. There is also a balance between focusing on discussion about "therapy" rather than on the person's current immediate concerns and needs. The sooner you can enable the person to take the lead in discussing what concerns him- or herself, the better. This will limit the amount of introductory discussion provided, but at a later stage more description of what therapy involves may be possible.

The introduction might begin (for example):

> "Hello, I'm [name]. Your doctor asked me to see you to see if there's any way I can be of help. She's given me some details, but do you want to start off by telling me how you see things?"

Phrasing such as "What problems do you have?" may not work with a person who is already alienated from others, especially if he or she is antagonistic toward official agencies and individuals. The response may be a hostile "I've got no problems. . . . Are you saying all this is my fault?" "How do you feel?"—with someone who is angry—may get the response "Well, how would you feel if the same things had happened to you?" If in doubt, take a neutral approach as above, but adapting your introduction to take account of the individual's needs and attitudes is important.

Explicit discussion of cognitive therapy may occur as part of a general discussion of what you, as a mental health worker, may have to offer, or it may be the sole focus of the work that you are likely to do as a therapist. It may be appropriate to discuss right at the start: the person may ask "Well, how can you help me?" Or as the initial assessment comes to a close, a discussion of where your sessions should go next will naturally lead on to such a discussion.

A "layered" explanation may be most appropriate—for many, simply the fact that you are seeing the person and allowing him or her to talk freely is most important.

"What we'll do, if it's OK with you, is meet for a few times to talk through what's been happening to you and see how much sense we can make of it. And maybe we can look at what might be done about it."

It may be that the "few times" is defined or you wish to define it, for example, "for five sessions and then we'll review." It may be necessary for service reasons (e.g., related to remuneration or contract definition) to establish a set number of sessions. It may also give a structure to therapy that can be helpful to clients. At the same time, there is some advantage in not predetermining length with them until it has become clearer how long is appropriate and possible. If, after assessment, it looks likely that you'll need to meet regularly over a few months, that may well be sufficient to say. It is, of course, essential that you be able to review the number and frequency of sessions needed. But if this can be done session by session, rather than necessarily in set blocks, the flexibility allowed can have advantages in adapting to the person's rate of change and needs as well as improving the efficiency of the service you can offer generally.

The person may want more information or feel he or she needs to understand more about cognitive therapy at this stage. In this case, you could say something like:

"You've been referred to me because I am trained [or am being trained] in using a specific approach to help people with the type of problems that you have, called cognitive therapy. It's a way of understanding how thoughts, feelings and behavior link together and that can be very helpful in disentangling and dealing with distressing experiences, like the voices you're hearing [or concerns you have]."

If you think it possible that the person has heard of cognitive therapy, you may want to explore that and elicit their preconceptions of it: "Have you ever heard of cognitive therapy? What have you heard?" But most people presenting with psychosis will not have. They may feel embarrassed at not knowing about cognitive therapy or puzzled that you are using an "obscure" therapy. Therefore, unless asked, we tend to normalize language and simply talk about helping them with their problems. It may be useful to provide reading material where further information is relevant and wanted (see Appendix 4, leaflet titled "Cognitive Therapy of Psychosis").

Choices about which type of therapy or specific techniques may be available to the person (including medication, cognitive therapy, or other intervention) need to be discussed. It may be appropriate to say at an early stage what your skills and expertise are. Some of this may be implicit; for example, if you are a psychologist, psychiatrist, nurse social worker, or community mental health counselor, the person will have certain expectations shaped by what the referrer has said and the person's general knowledge, experience, and understanding. At some stage, it may be important to explore these expectations. You may need to explain that you are trained or are training in cognitive therapy primarily or in addition to your professional training and that this will shape the assessment and formulation you make. But also say that you will consider other options, for example, medication or other forms of psychotherapy, and either provide them yourself, if trained and able to do so, or discuss referral to someone who can make an appropriate assessment and provide appropriate care.

Cognitive therapy now has a strong evidence base in psychosis, especially with persistent symptoms, and this is increasingly being supported by official sources. It is important to provide details of this evidence if the person wants to know more, but for many the following statement is sufficient:

"Cognitive therapy has been investigated thoroughly, and the evidence for its help-ing with the sort of persistent problems you have is now good. That doesn't mean that it works for everyone, but we can expect it to be of, at least some help."

With people presenting for the first time with symptoms of psychosis or sugges-tive of psychosis, the evidence currently is more limited. However, it is reasonable to say:

"Cognitive therapy has been investigated thoroughly for the sort of problems you have and is effective when the problems have been present for a while. We are still investigating whether it works as well when problems are just beginning. But we can expect it to be at least of some help."

There are alternative or complementary options, especially the use of medication, which have a well-developed evidence base. There are also therapies such as Hogarty's Personal Therapy (Hogarty et al., 1997) and psychodynamic therapies for which some evidence of effectiveness exists. But the latter, in particular, has yet to be shown to be ef-fective for psychosis, using the generally accepted ways, such as by randomized con-trolled trial. The former—in the study that has been published—seemed effective for people living with caregivers but not those living alone. This is not to say that these therapies and also complementary therapies, such as aromatherapy, are not helpful; it is just that they have not been clearly demonstrated to be so. Some people and thera-pists do think that there are benefits to them, but most health systems do not fund their use. Psychodynamic therapy, which generally involves interpretations being made, contrasts with cognitive therapy, where collaboration is used to arrive at understanding of problems, and this makes their use in combination or in parallel difficult, as the dif-fering approaches are probably too confusing to the person and counterproductive. So, if the person wants and can obtain psychodynamic therapy, it is probably best to discontinue formal cognitive therapy until that therapy is completed or discontinued itself. It is still of course possible to use collaborative techniques with the use of medica-tion and other psychosocial interventions, for example, vocational and other rehabilita-tion.

Some people may wish to discontinue medication and participate in cognitive therapy as an alternative. Our stance has been that medication seems to have beneficial effects for at least 70–80% of people with schizophrenia, and so we strongly advocate it in appropriate dosage. It is not possible currently to identify which people with schizo-phrenia will not respond, and so currently medication is recommended for all. Risks with the newer antipsychotics are generally low, although caution is needed, especially with clozapine. All the studies that have been described earlier advocate the combina-tion of cognitive therapy with adequate medication, and so we know this to be an effec-tive option. We do not know whether cognitive therapy used alone has any effects be-cause there are no studies available currently using cognitive therapy alone as an alternative to medication. Undertaking such a study could prove difficult and cause ethical concerns, although there might be a place for such a study among people who refuse medication. However, there are quite a few people who do refuse medication or who discontinue it during therapy. Offering or continuing with cognitive therapy seems reasonable and may help them see the potential benefits of a combined medication and therapy approach.

Some people—for example, those with persistent abusive hallucinations—will refuse medication because they can see no evidence of benefit to themselves but can see, often supported by their relatives, obvious side effects of the medication. On an individual basis, we will often provide continuing support to them despite their not taking medication. We have worked with a substantial number of people with whom we have eventually agreed that for them—because they have remained well over a number of years—a drug-free existence is a reasonable one to choose; but we do not advocate this. More commonly, negotiating to reduce levels of medication is appropriate, and assisting the person in making his or her case to the prescriber can be a valuable part of therapy, assisting both the prescriber and the recipient.

There are potential issues surrounding whether the role of the therapist can be simultaneously combined with that of case manager, nurse, psychologist, or psychiatrist. In some cases these roles might conflict, while in others the combination might enhance the treatment. With severe mental illnesses there are frequently occasions when combining roles seems helpful, such as:

- When adherence to a management plan (including taking medication or attending a social group) is proving difficult for the person.
- When engagement is a problem and assistance with financial or accommodation issues (by advocacy to others or through the therapist's role as case manager) can promote it.
- When relating to one individual rather than many may help and the person may insist on it (that is, being both therapist and psychiatrist or case manager may be requested or demanded by the person).
- When continuity of care may be promoted, as, for example, the therapist may remain in contact with the person as case manager even when therapy, as such, has ended (but can be restarted if needed).

Alternatively, there may be circumstances in which the roles conflict. For the therapist who is also a case manager or psychiatrist:

- He or she may have to use involuntary measures to hospitalize the client or ensure that medication is taken.
- There may be personality clashes.
- Sufficient time for therapy may not be available.
- Time protected from other commitments (e.g., being on call or subject to interruptions) may be difficult to establish.

For the therapist who is only a therapist:

- Working without conflicts over medication and the like may allow work to proceed that otherwise would be affected.
- Dedicated time or a regular basis that is uninterrupted by other demands may be easier to establish.

In summary, orientation of clients to treatment involves much more than simply describing what the therapy is to them. It involves understanding what they understand about therapy—their preconceptions about it. It is about helping them develop new ways of looking at what has happened to them and what *can* happen. It also involves describing the options available and negotiating with them over agreement to proceed and even areas of therapy that are acceptable. For example, many clients agree to participate as long as certain issues, often related to traumatic experiences, are not discussed. Agreement to this can allow a relationship to develop that in time may enable the client to talk about matters previously "off limits."

The language used and the method of conveying what cognitive therapy may have to offer them is an important part of engaging clients in therapy. If the explanation is too technical or given in a way that seems to them irrelevant to their needs, they may not be prepared to work with you. Their decision to become involved may be influenced by providing evidence that this is a therapy that has been effective with people with similar problems to their own. Such evidence may be provided by description or written evidence—even copies of review articles—if the person wishes.

ORIENTING THE CLIENT TO TREATMENT

Gordon (*sensitivity psychosis***)**: Discussion of cognitive therapy was accepted without difficulty early on in the sessions by Gordon, who was keen to look at alternatives to medication but eventually accepted that the combination of therapy with medication was most likely to be efficacious.

Craig (*drug-related psychosis***)**: Talking about cognitive therapy was more complicated, and a more formal approach seemed to be rejected by Craig, who was unwilling for a number of years to engage in any psychological intervention. This was also exacerbated by persistent thought disorder. Eventually an approach that simply stressed understanding what was happening to him and emphasized finding ways to cope and reduce the severity of his symptoms was accepted by him, such that he attended regularly for sessions and participated actively in therapy.

Gillian (*traumatic psychosis***)**: Introducing a new way of helping Gillian was part of the engagement process. She was frightened and had limited ability to comprehend even a simple explanation of cognitive therapy because of the distraction of her symptoms and limited intelligence. Explaining that the therapist intended to help by allowing her to talk about what had happened to her and see if they could work out ways of making this better—especially the voices—was the limit of the initial orientation process. As time passed, slightly more sophisticated concepts—for example, linking current symptoms and memories to past events—became possible.

Paul (*anxiety psychosis***)**: The major issue in explaining the cognitive model to Paul was to avoid disengagement. He could perfectly well understand the concepts but might easily object to such a conceptualization: "so, you don't believe me, then. You are saying it's my thoughts that are the problems. You think this is all in my mind." Assessment and formulation therefore progressed on the basis of an agreement that understanding what had happened to him would be the first step in working together. At a later stage, as Paul himself began to make links between thoughts and behavior, the model was gradually introduced.

EIGHT

Psychoeducation and Normalization

The key to the client's being able to understand the distressing and confusing experiences that occur in schizophrenia is psychoeducation based on the case formulation. This involves providing or, better still, eliciting from the person him- or herself psychological explanations for the symptoms. For example:

> Harold felt pressure on his head that he believed was generated by an external force. Discussion of how anxiety can cause tension in the neck muscles, which have an effect on connecting muscles radiating upward—causing a feeling of pressure—provided an alternative explanation that he was prepared to consider.

A specific form of psychoeducation is normalization, in which symptoms—such as voices and paranoia—that appear to be "abnormal" and associated with "madness" are discussed. These are compared with the experiences described by normal volunteers in, for example, sleep or sensory deprivation experiments or by people subjected to unusual forms of stress (e.g., people taken hostage) or just feeling oversensitive (e.g., fleeting paranoid feelings on entering a room that seems to go quiet as you enter, immediately prompting the thought "Were they talking about *me*?").

PSYCHOEDUCATION

Psychoeducation has for many years been a key feature of therapeutic programs. There is good evidence that it is a valuable tool in helping clients, and their caregivers, to know what's wrong with them, what diagnosis they have, and how the condition may have developed. For any illness, whether depression, diabetes, or cancer, such information is helpful. But especially with schizophrenia—such a stigmatized disorder that is constantly being linked with aggression and poor prognosis—it is crucial for clients to have a clear understanding of what is known about the illness and what is myth or supposition. However, psychoeducation about schizophrenia has also been associated with an increase in suicidal thinking (Cunningham-Owens et al., 2001). An increase in acceptance of illness, in our own work, has also been associated not with improved overall symptom outcome, as is insight overall, but with increased depression (Rathod et al., 2003). It is for this reason that we have suggested that psychoeducation needs to be embedded in a cognitive-behavioral framework and that careful consideration needs to be given to its use, especially emphasis upon the use of the diagnostic term "schizophrenia." Unfortunately, the erroneous associations with this term have led us to be very careful in using it and also to seek out relevant related or alternative expressions such as sensitivity, trauma, anxiety, and drug-related conditions, and to develop literature (and ongoing research) to support this approach (see the leaflet titled "What's the Problem?" in Appendix 4).

Individualizing psychoeducation helps people feel listened to and understood, and this approach adds to its effectiveness. Early on during the assessment process, such questions as these should be asked:

- "What would you like to know about what has happened to you?"
- "How has it been described to you previously?"
- "How did you feel about that?"
- "What did it mean to you?"

If the person is not aware of their diagnosis, feels uneasy, or rejects it, we do not continue to emphasize it.

Three components of insight have been delineated (David, 1990). The client may

- Accept the need for treatment.
- Accept that he or she has an illness.
- Accept that voices or delusions are originating from within him- or herself.

There is evidence that increased acceptance of the need for treatment and recognition that the voices or delusions are originating from within oneself both correlate positively with improved outcomes. It seems reasonable therefore to focus on these matters. Whenever descriptive terms are needed, the names of the four subgroups identified earlier are used. Conditions related to stress sensitivity, drugs, past trauma, and anxiety, seem relatively easy for people to accept. Discussions about whether they have "schizophrenia" are potentially damaging to engagement and therapy. The most important consideration is that they have problems that may benefit from collaboration with mental health services and the treatment options available.

Whatever the client's attitude toward a diagnosis of schizophrenia, what is key is the person's acceptance that he or she is unwell, "stressed," or just that things are "not right." In that context, some education about known vulnerability factors and interaction with stressful events is invaluable. However, as described previously (in Chapters 2 and 6), this information is probably better imparted as an explanation of the client's own vulnerability factors and stressors rather than as a separate and rather theoretical exposition. Opportunities for people with schizophrenia and their caregivers to read, watch videos, go to talks, or discuss their beliefs about the illness with each other may be useful in supplementing this education. However, in individual work—which this manual is most concerned with—individual discussion based on the person's circumstances and symptoms remains the most effective way of providing appropriate education.

Describing the client's vulnerabilities, strengths, and stressors to him or her may be highly instructive:

> "Why do people develop illnesses of the type that you have? Simply, this is the result of things happening to them that they feel to be stressful, causing them to hear voices or develop strong beliefs that to them seem to explain what is happening. Of course, stress doesn't usually do this to people, so we think it occurs where or when people are vulnerable in some way. So, they may have a family history of similar problems or a particularly sensitive personality. It is possible that there are changes in the brain that make people vulnerable, but it remains unclear as to what these might be. Isolation, sleep disturbance, and use of some drugs are also possible factors. Some people are more vulnerable than others and need less stress to become ill; for others, the stress may be colossal before they develop the sort of symptoms that you have."

It remains very important to have a collaborative discussion about this, checking what has been understood, what has been agreed with or disagreed with. You may want to go on further to discuss the secondary effects of illness:

> "As stress decreases, so recovery may occur, but unfortunately sometimes becoming ill has meant that other stresses have developed, as seems to have happened with you . . . [It is best to use a personally relevant example.] For example, you may have lost your job, or relationships may have been affected. It may have affected how you and sometimes, unfortunately, others think about yourself. All this can make it more difficult for you to get back to how things were before you became ill."

Education that normalizes appropriately can be highly valued. The use of technical terms can be off-putting if they are not explained fully to the person and should be used only when simpler alternatives would not be effective. However, there is a place for developing their use by clients to better understand their experiences, give them a name, and in the process be able to distance themselves from them. This can allow them to analyze the experiences more objectively; for example, some of our clients have developed the use of such terms as "somatic hallucinations," "paranoia," and "thought broadcasting" to describe these phenomena themselves, and this has been accompanied by improved insight into them.

Discussion of medication and other treatment interventions is also frequently necessary (e.g., orienting the client to cognitive therapy, as discussed previously). The influence of the therapist over prescribed medications can vary from nil to total control (as the doctor or where legislation allows it, clinical psychologist or nurse). If the therapist has no direct control, the client's understanding of the potential effects of medication and its side effects in psychosis is well worth developing. Medications can moderate or eliminate symptoms, but frequently continuing prophylaxis is needed to prevent recurrence. But for how long? This will depend on individual factors, and discussion with the prescriber may be helpful to establish his or her views of this. There is considerable variation in the prescribing regimes used and in the responses by recipients. Although often very helpful, some people are not demonstrably helped by medication, but the decision to take them off it totally is a difficult one for most prescribers to make. There is often the belief that medication is unlikely to do much harm but may be having some benefit (even if it is difficult to detect) or potential to prevent deterioration (even from a very distressed and disabled state). However, side effects can include sedation, weight gain, tremors, restlessness, rigidity, and a variety of other effects, even with the group of drugs introduced during the past decade.[1]

The reasons why these drugs are effective on psychotic symptoms has been the subject of much research but remains controversial. However, all those that are effective have an action on dopamine, although individual drugs also affect other chemicals in the brain. Dopamine produces noradrenaline and in turn adrenaline—it forms part of a "stress pathway," and we tend to describe it as this to people who wish to know. From its effect on reducing relapse, it seems reasonable that it is "buffering" individuals against stress or whatever it is that precipitates relapse. When medication has sedative effects, it can also assist with sleep and anxiety. So, a simple explanation might be:

> "We're not sure exactly why these drugs are effective. But they all seem to act on a chemical called dopamine, which forms part of a 'stress pathway.' They seem to 'buffer' against stress and can assist with sleep and anxiety and also voices and disturbing beliefs."

Some people want more information and will search books and the Internet for further guidance. Providing information up to the level they require—and perhaps a little more—is well appreciated. The person may want reductions or increases in medication—or to discontinue it altogether. In the end, it is the person who takes the medication who gains any potential benefits and experiences any adverse effects, and only rarely are there risks to others in the person's not taking that medication. It is easy to reach a point of disagreement—"I think you need this medication and without it you will become ill again [or get much worse]" versus "But I don't want to take it"—that may not be said explicitly but is acted upon. It is easy for the mental health practitioner to become authoritarian and the client frustrated. The evidence seems to support a willingness to negotiate as being most successful in the long run, though short-term risk considerations may also come into play. Going through the process described below may avoid the necessity of resorting to involuntary measures and favorably shape the client's attitudes toward future discussions of the issue.

> "OK, so I understand that you do not want to take any medication." Could we try discussing the range of drugs available that I think might help you and what doses are possible?
>
> > "There are four or five drugs [*list names*] we could look at—you've tried a couple of them. How did you get on with them?
> >
> > "The effects of each of them are similar. They do have different additional effects—some which can be a benefit and some which are side effects. For example,

---

[1]Drugs have proprietary names given to them by the companies producing them and generic—chemical—names as well. The newer group of antipsychotic drugs includes olanzepine, risperidone, quetiapine, amisulpride, aripiprazole, ziprasidone, and zotepine. Older drugs include chlorpromazine, thorazine, haloperidol, trifluoperazine, and sulpiride. Finally, clozapine is a drug used in people who have not responded to any of the aforementioned drugs.

[drug A] helps more with sleep and agitation. [You may then give a brief explanation of common effects—this could be supplemented with written information. The person may then want time to consider this, during the interview preferably but may need to go away and return at a later stage.]

"Are there any of these drugs that you would prefer? [You may want to discuss this further.]

"We need to consider dosage. If we look at your previous experience with medication this may help. [It may be that a negotiation occurs that results in the person being on dosages lower than you would recommend, but you can agree to 'see how it goes' and 'keep it under review.']"

Sometimes the person refuses medication altogether, despite the risk considerations:

"OK, we are not going to agree. Let's see how things go without medication. Could we discuss what you need to look out for that might suggest that things are going downhill? [Discuss relapse prevention—see Chapter 14.]

"Or simply if your symptoms [voices, paranoia, etc.] are getting worse, could you get in touch with me rapidly and we can review the situation?

"Otherwise, could we meet in [e.g., 1, 2, 4] weeks time?"

This leaves the door open for the client to return, as we find they often do, if problems develop. And sometimes they are right: medication is not necessary, and they remain well without it—even though we may consider that the risks to groups of people with their particular problems favor their taking it. If these discussions end in disagreement, it is that much more difficult for people to return and reassess the situation. They are also more likely to deny to themselves that they are becoming ill or worsening.

Caregivers, both families and mental health staff, may find this way of working challenging, and you may have to spend time explaining why you are not commanding the person to do as he or she is told—rather, you are negotiating with another human being who has the right to make decisions about what chemicals he or she ingests. The rights of the caregivers may also enter the picture, but essentially such evidence as there is—and our experience certainly confirms this—suggests much more favorable outcomes with a negotiated way of proceeding.

"NORMALIZATION" OF PSYCHOSIS

Much of what we aim to do has its roots in a philosophy of care that recognizes that people experiencing psychotic illnesses are not different types of people from ourselves, although they may be having experiences that are unlike those that we have had. Even the latter qualification may just be a question of degree rather than type.

Normalization is the process by which thoughts, behaviors, moods, and experiences are compared and understood in terms of similar thoughts, behaviors, moods, and experiences attributed to other individuals who are *not* diagnosed as ill—especially mentally ill (see Table 8.1). These experiences are usually related to some form of stress, but often the difference between whether they seriously distress or interfere with

TABLE 8.1. **Aims of Normalization**

- To promote understanding of psychological phenomena that also resemble symptoms of schizophrenia
- To reduce "fear of going mad"
- To facilitate:
  —Reattribution of hallucinations
  —Alternative explanations of delusions
- To improve self-esteem
- To reduce isolation and feelings of isolation
- To reduce stigma:
  —By others: family, friends, neighbors, general public
  —By self

people's lives only temporarily or rather worsen to become longer-term illnesses is that they are not sufficiently well understood as being primarily stress-related. For example, hostages may experience hallucinations or paranoia while captive but will usually understand this as being caused by their situation. After being released, they may still have distress related to the experience but do not usually go on to develop "schizophrenia," as they properly attribute their distress to their previous time as a hostage.

Hearing your name called when you are tired, although nobody seems to have called it (an example of "hyponogogic hallucinations"), or walking into a noisy room that suddenly goes quiet and wondering whether people had been talking about you are attenuated (or near) examples of psychotic symptoms. That such fleeting experiences do not persist as an ongoing problem and are recognized for what they are distinguishes psychiatric from nonpsychiatric belief. But the phenomena nonetheless remain on a continuum with psychosis. Much of this knowledge is "common sense" but often not applied where it can be most useful—in understanding perplexing situations and perceptions. The use of guided discovery with the client can draw out his or her own understanding and knowledge:

"Have you heard of any other circumstances where people have gotten confused or heard voices? . . . What would you expect to happen to somebody who was deprived of sleep for several days? Or left isolated in a room for several weeks?"

This usually needs supplementing but can often open up useful routes to explore.

Understanding the Effects on Individuals of Stigmatization and Discrimination

Normalization is such an important concept because of its influence on stigmatization and discrimination against people who are experiencing or even have previously experienced psychoses. Such stigmatization can occur:

- By others—strangers and even friends encountered in neighborhoods, workplaces, hospitals, and so on
- By therapists
- By family members and caregivers
- By the person themselves—effects on self-esteem and expectations

Psychoses, especially schizophrenia, have classically been viewed as "different" from other conditions, both physical and even mental. Much of the distress and disability experienced by people with psychoses can be attributed to precisely this phenomenon. It may be part of the reason why people with schizophrenia in the "developed world" are considered to have a worse prognosis than others. Much of this fear or worry may have to do with the typical difficulty in understanding people with these problems; after all, thought disorders may cloud or confuse communications, and much of what such persons say "doesn't seem to make sense." Persons with schizophrenia may therefore act in unpredictable ways and cause people to fear that such actions may involve aggression toward them—a fear exacerbated by the media.

People with psychoses may be stigmatized by neighbors or workmates, thereby increasing the stress experienced and paranoia felt. In medical centers, similar fears can mean that normally requisite physical investigations are not performed, contributing to a higher illness and death rate within this group. It also seems likely that such mass opprobrium has had the effect of diminishing resources devoted to services for those with schizophrenia, as well as research into their problems. Even families and caregivers may be influenced by the exaggerated or erroneous information dispensed by the media and others such that it can cause them unnecessary fear and even estrangement from the individual, although usually the knowledge of the person as an individual—the personal relationship—counteracts this.

The term "schizophrenia" is often accompanied by fears of unpredictability, embarrassment, violence, and inevitable deterioration in the future. The aim of destigmatization is to reduce these fears and misunderstandings and the consequent guilt, hostility, and criticism to which they can give rise.

At its root is this belief that people with psychoses are "different," and yet there is substantial research demonstrating otherwise (e.g., Oswald, 1974; Leff, 1968). Understanding the nature of this research can be valuable for the person, the caregivers, and others in "normalizing" these experiences. The one proviso that needs consideration is that the suggestion that people with schizophrenia or psychosis "are like us—only more so" could play into fears that individuals have of themselves going "mad," thereby leading to exacerbation of those fears and, indeed, active resistance to the idea of a continuum.

Normalization directed at therapists and mental health professionals is also beneficial. Schizophrenia and psychosis have long been viewed as "beyond therapy." This is because of evidence from clinical studies during the 1960s and 1970s of the ineffectiveness of psychodynamic approaches, a perception of schizophrenia as being only likely to respond to biological approaches and, from "Jaspers onward" (i.e., from early in the 20th century onwards), the "non-understandability" of it. With evidence for the effectiveness of treatments (described previously) and the potential for understanding the experiences that people describe, it is time that psychosis and schizophrenia be accepted as "normal" mental disorders—sometimes difficult to treat but on a continuum with other illnesses (see Figure 5.1 on p. 63).

Understanding the Effects of Specific Stressors in Producing Psychotic Symptoms

So, normalizing therapists' reactions to clients' recounting of their experiences or display of behavior is an important start. We use such normalizing with other mental health difficulties. For example, explanations of chest pain occurring in panic disorder may invoke analogies with pain that can occur in other circumstances for reasons other than illness (e.g., "cramps" with exercise, or headaches). In borderline personality disorder, self-harm—"overdosing" with medication, substance misuse, or cutting oneself—can be difficult to understand until it is recognized just how highly effective these ways are of reducing acute distress in the short term even though they may be risky and damaging activities especially in the long term.

In relation to psychosis, there are numerous situations in which specific stresses can cause symptoms of psychosis. Some of these are experimental, others due to unusual but understandable circumstances. As described, deprivation states are classic examples where normal volunteers deprived of sleep or sensation will develop a range of perceptions that become more and more distorted as time passes and with the intensity of the deprivation. Sensory deprivation experiments during the 1960s produced perceptions in subjects ranging from mild distortions and unease to symptoms that in other circumstances could be described as diagnostic of schizophrenia. Where the deprivation was greatest (e.g., using water-tanks and complete darkness), these experiences were the most intense and came on the most rapidly. Experiments with medical students in which they were deprived of sleep led to some of them becoming irritable, paranoid, hallucinated, and exhibiting bizarre behavior. However, because these experiments were part of experimental situations and so could be terminated on immediate request from the subjects and also understandable to those monitoring them and the subjects themselves, it can be expected that full "recovery" occurred, although a stressful event of this type in someone vulnerable could potentially persist or the perceptions recur—as memories do ("flashbacks"). Posttraumatic stress disorder presents with phenomena that are similar to psychotic symptoms—"flashbacks" can be very similar to hallucinations but, because they are accepted by the person concerned as internal phenomena (i.e., their own experiences), they are not "psychotic" phenomena. As described earlier, this appears to be on a continuum with psychosis ("posttraumatic stress psychosis"), and people may drift across the line into and back out of psychosis readily. Other circumstances that may be relevant (see Table 8.2), for example, hostage situations, can lead to people developing "psychotic" symptoms, although there is certainly a case to be made that these are appropriate adaptations to extreme circumstances. There are a number of biographies detailing these (e.g., Brian Keenan [1992] in *An Evil Cradling* describing vivid visual hallucinations).

There are also "delusional" beliefs that are comparable to psychotic ones. The

---

TABLE 8.2. "Normal" Circumstances in Which Psychotic Symptoms Can Occur

- Deprivation states—sleep, sensory, etc.
- Fear—for example, hostage situations
- Trauma—for example, associated with PTSD and sexual and physical abuse
- Organic—for example, drug-induced, other toxic, fever, and drug or alcohol withdrawal states, brain stimulation
- Bereavement—misidentification and hallucinatory phenomena
- Hypnogogic and hypnopompic hallucinations (immediately before and after sleep)
- Trance states—for example, in religious ceremonies

Note. Reviewed in Kingdon and Turkington (1994).

TABLE 8.3. Belief in "Unscientific" Phenomena

68%	God
>50%	Thought transference
>50%	Predicting future events
>25%	Ghosts
25%	Superstitions
25%	Reincarnation
23%	Horoscopes
21%	The devil

Note. Data from Cox and Cowling (1989).

oversensitivity to others (described earlier), even if fleeting in nature, compares with the persistent experience of paranoia. The importance of other people's confirmation or denial of suspicions cannot be overemphasized. If, after walking into a room that suddenly goes quiet, someone already in the room tells you that the assembled were not, in fact, talking about you—and you trust that person to tell you the truth—that will generally be enough to dismiss the idea—unless it is reinforced by some other incident. If you fear somebody is following you in the street, checking with a trustworthy partner what the evidence for this was can either supply reassurance for your suspicions or a way to check it out, for example, that person can watch you leave and see if anyone follows you. If no one can do this for you or be there to discuss these concerns, it is conceivable that they are more likely to take root and a self-confirming bias—whereby you may begin to interpret evidence in a way that supports your worst fears—will take over.

Belief in various "nonscientific" phenomena is very common. Relating psychotic symptoms to such phenomena can be a very effective way of opening them to rational argument. It can also provide a common language and assist in your engaging with the client. Table 8.3 provides a summary of the level of belief in such phenomena, demonstrating how common it is. For some, such beliefs are comforting and help explain their world; others believe that such phenomena seriously interfere with their lives and potentially the lives of others as, for example, the alleged dependence of a U.S. president's wife (Nancy Reagan) on horoscopes. The fear of ghosts and the devil may also be a significant component of some people's lives. But, of course, most people in those circumstances are not described as psychotic. The distinction between "beliefs" and "delusions" appears to be primarily socially determined. Beliefs that are properly described as delusions are:

- Strongly held
- Understandable (but only once the context is fully appreciated)
- Not agreed to by family, friends, or companions—at least to the extent held to be true by the person concerned
- In the exceptional case of a "folie-à-deux," similar beliefs are shared by two family members or spouses living together

Some specific beliefs may be useful in tackling psychotic symptoms—for example, reconceptualizing thought broadcasting as telepathy or passivity as hypnosis or another form of external control such as magnetism (see Chapter 11). In all such circumstances, normalization seems to assist by promoting self-esteem, reducing the feeling of estrangement from others, and appropriately reattributing experiences that may seem externally generated to internal causes.

Risks of Normalizing

The greatest risk of normalizing may be the untoward minimizing of problems—at the extreme, "Oh, we all hear voices—so what's your problem?" More generally, the acceptance of hearing voices might be taken to mean that you just have to get on and live with them. It may well be that, given sufficient or specific stresses to which we are all vulnerable, it is probable that anyone can develop psychotic beliefs. Such stresses might include being poisoned, for example, by hallucinogenic drugs, or being physically ill with delirium. Nevertheless, the experiences themselves can be extremely distressing, especially if they can't be understood or the only conceivable explanation to the person most concerned is a very disturbing one—to wit, "The Mafia is poisoning me—they think I owe them money!"

The risks of normalizing therefore include minimizing or failing to deal with consequences or the development of the belief that

> "If it's not my illness, I must be bad" or "If it's me thinking this rather than someone outside saying it, I must really be evil!"

As described later, this belief, once identified, can be worked with successfully, but first it needs to be identified—and it may be, thanks to normalizing explanations.

Automatic Thoughts

One subject that can cause serious misunderstanding is the concept of automatic thoughts. Although a universal phenomenon, automatic thoughts are not one that is widely understood. Moreover the introspection that occurs when people are depressed or confused can lead to major distressing connotations being attached to their "automatic thoughts." However, fully understanding automatic thoughts may help clients to make the key distinction between thoughts and actions, which is central to the cognitive model of schizophrenia and other emotional disorders.

When clients are confused about their own thoughts, perhaps presenting with a jumble of psychotic beliefs or voices, the thoughts or voices may be negative and viewed as true "because I wouldn't think it otherwise"—or, alternatively, they may be mundane but not accepted as the person's own thoughts sometimes "because they seem so stupid." A general explanation may prove instructive:

> "Perhaps it would help if we just talked a little bit about the way thoughts happen. Often they seem to be something we control: we decide to look at a newspaper and read it—leading us to think about it. Or we may be talking and thinking about what we are saying. But much of the time our thoughts go on, whatever we're doing or concentrating on. For example, while we're chatting here, I expect you'll have had a thought like "I really would like a glass of water or a cup of coffee" or

"I wonder how long this is going to go on" or "What is he talking about?" Does that make sense? Do you know the sorts of thoughts that I mean?"

Most people seem to recognize this layer of thoughts that goes on automatically when demonstrated in this way—particularly if it is made relevant to the situation. For example, if a truck were loudly driven past the interview room, "That was noisy" would be a reasonable comment in passing. A further way to help clients recognize automatic thoughts is to get them to think about what happens when they go to bed to sleep. As one is lying down waiting for sleep to come, one's mind will flow through events of the day and will often focus on particularly significant concerns. This flow of thoughts is automatic, with some occasional redirection, and can be a good illustration that also can highlight key concerns that the person has. "What are you thinking about when you are trying to get to sleep?" often identifies key issues in people with all forms of mental health problems, including psychoses.

The automatic nature of thoughts can be discussed, describing how triggers—like a specific word or sight—can be associated with significant events or people and then thoughts flow in that direction. It may also be relevant to discuss thoughts' association with mood. When one is depressed, thoughts also tend to be negative (and, similarly, negative thoughts may lead to a depressed mood). A particular issue is the intrusion of aggressive, hostile, or sexual thoughts or just ones that are strange. The simple occurrence of these may lead to the person's accusing him- or herself of being bad or mad— "How could I think something like that?"—especially in relation to a specific person, for example, a child or parent. The belief underlying this is that if you think something it must indicate that "subconsciously" it is something that you might wish to do or be made to do (even against your will). Explanation of the "flow of consciousness" can be illuminating and reduce self-castigation (i.e., that it is "not your fault" that your thoughts have pursued such a direction). These thoughts are often obsessional in nature. But there is a relative lack of literature to provide supporting descriptions of this—Molly Bloom's soliloquy in James Joyce's *Ulysses* is probably the best literary example of automatic thoughts. Work on intrusive thoughts in obsessive–compulsive disorder also uses similar normalizing principles. For example, there are excellent descriptions of the thoughts and impulses of nonclinical samples (Rachman & de Silva, 1978). These individuals describe spontaneous thoughts of, for example, intense anger toward someone, of harm to or the death of a family member, and of acts of violence in sex. Similarly, impulses to say something nasty and damning to someone; to hurt or harm them; to jump on the tracks when a subway train is approaching; to physically and verbally attack someone; to harm or be violent toward children, especially smaller ones; to crash cars when driving; and to attack and violently punish someone—for example, to throw a child out of a bus. Relevant self-disclosure may be the most effective way to proceed in confirming these "normal thoughts" and in normalizing them, as it can reinforce the message given:

"There's nothing stranger than the thoughts that can go through your mind."

Thoughts may also be "disowned." That is, they can be transformed from being *obsessional* to being *psychotic* whenever the person "disowns them"—as voices or thoughts inserted into his or her mind.

"They couldn't be *my* thoughts. I couldn't possibly think something like *that*."

Similarly, voices, as they are reattributed to self during treatment or simply the progress of the illness, become obsessions in many circumstances, especially when the content is negative.

Something else important to normalize is the relationship between thoughts and actions. Essentially this involves being able to distinguish a thought from an intent to do something and subsequently an action based on it. Thoughts are not actions—they may lead to them, but only if the person wishes or allows them to happen. For example, you think you would like a cup of coffee, and so you go and make one. However, you may think of harming yourself or someone else (as described above in nonclinical samples) but can reject that thought and not act upon it. The feeling of compulsion may be strong, and a psychotic belief in control from outside can further complicate this picture, but, as discussed later (in Chapter 11), retaining personal responsibility for actions is reinforced by discussion of the distinction between thoughts and actions (see Table 8.4).

Decatastrophization

Much of what has been described in this chapter aims to decatastrophize fears that have developed from strange, worrisome, or confusing experiences. Essentially the objective is to avoid "making a catastrophe out of a crisis" or, whenever the catastrophe seems to be occurring, help the person to reevaluate what is happening to him or her in such a way that the person understands it better, engages in self-blame less, and is welcomed back as an equal member of the human race.

The subjective fear of "going crazy" is the most frequent symptom of such an event (Hirsch & Jolley, 1989)

PSYCHOEDUCATION AND NORMALIZATION

Gordon (*sensitivity psychosis*): Gaining his acceptance that he had mental health problems and his agreement to take medication took some time with Gordon, especially since his parents were also unconvinced. But, as time has passed, he now

---

TABLE 8.4. **Using Normalization**

- Use for engagement.
- Normalize, don't minimize.
- Use with guided discovery.
- Use a conversational style.
- Reinforce the person's own functional beliefs.
- Don't neglect suggestions from the person, a caregiver, or others.
- But beware the response isn't "You must think I'm nuts!"—perhaps use phrases such as "Some people believe in . . . "
- But how far do you go in saying "this is normal?"
- How do you know? How much are you influenced by your own beliefs?
- Normalize settings and environments.
- Use community teams visiting at home or based in the locality.
- Improve environments, decor, etc.
- Use simple self-help—for example, reading relevant literature.

understands himself to have schizophrenia. This has become a particular issue now in terms of how he describes what has been wrong with him to employers. We have agreed on an approach that gives minimal but accurate information in the first instance, for example, avoiding the term "schizophrenia" because of its stigma and using "anxiety" or "depression" (which he has also experienced), with further details to be supplied by his medical practitioner when requested. Particular normalization techniques that were used included discussion of "sensitivity to stress" and a vulnerability–stress model; "telepathy" was also used to develop a common language in relation to his thought broadcasting.

Craig (*drug-related psychosis*): Psychoeducation was initially an issue with Craig, and discussion of drug use was complicated by continuing contact with friends who were using drugs. Normalization of symptoms through analogies, using dreams to understand voices and PTSD for the "flashbacks," has been valuable in developing the therapeutic relationship—which previously had proved impossible to establish.

Gillian (*traumatic psychosis*): Normalization has been invaluable in engaging with Gillian and in helping her begin to understand her voices. The simple idea that "not sleeping properly and getting stressed can make your mind play tricks on you" has made her symptoms more understandable. She has been told previously that she has schizophrenia, and since she had little understanding of what this meant at that time, she has not been particularly upset by it—but at the same time it has not made much of an impact on her understanding of her illness.

Paul (*anxiety psychosis*) : It was decided early on that psychoeducation using the term "schizophrenia" might lead Paul to reject the need for help and possibly disengage from services and noncollaborate on the need for medication. There were occasions when the term was mentioned by medical and other staff working with him, and he rejected the notion that he might be experiencing it. He did, however, accept that he had problems—that he was anxious—and the concept of an anxiety psychosis was one that he was prepared to discuss though not accept until considerable work had been done with his symptoms. Normalization material proved to be interesting to him—for example, the concept of brainwashing and other ways in which suggestibility can be induced.

NINE

Case Formulation and Intervening with Delusions

The traditional definition of a delusion effectively excluded the prospect of psychological remedies:

> A delusion is a false belief held with absolute certainty despite evidence to the contrary and out of keeping with the person's social, educational, cultural and religious background. (Hamilton, 1984)

There are a number of assumptions within this definition that are not supported by evidence: delusions often contain a kernel of truth and relate to premorbid interests and ideas (see review of the relevant literature in Kingdon & Turkington, 1994). Also, there are many bizarre unscientific beliefs held by a large proportion of the population—for example, beliefs in telepathy, poltergeists, alien abduction, and horoscopes (Kingdon et al., 1994)—that merge into "delusional" beliefs, and there is no distinct point at which they are not in keeping with the person's background. Furthermore, as demonstrated by the studies into the effectiveness of cognitive therapy, discussing the evidence without necessarily contradicting the client can lead to a change in the characteristics of the delusion. Redefining the traditional concept of "delusion" seems necessary to develop an understanding within psychiatry that psychological measures might be of benefit and that dichotomous views of psychopathology are not evidence-based (Strauss, 1969); that is, beliefs are a continuum between truth and falsehood.

The following evidence-based definition has been proposed (Turkington et al., 1996):

> A delusion is a belief (probably false) at the extreme end of the continuum of consensual agreement. It is not categorically different from overvalued ideas and normal beliefs. It is held in spite of evidence to the contrary but it may be amenable to change when that evidence is collaboratively explored. In that case the belief may come to approximate more closely to ideas in keeping with the person's social, cultural, educational and religious background.

Further, the belief may be fully understandable when the context in which it developed is known. This chapter looks at work with delusional beliefs in broad terms. Later chapters deal with more specific delusional beliefs as they relate to hallucinations, thought broadcasting, and "passivity" phenomena.

DEVISING AN INITIAL TREATMENT PLAN

In this section we describe how to develop a strategy for exploring and managing delusional beliefs through the development and use of the case formulation. Comprehensive assessment is the foundation from which a case formulation is built (see Chapter 5). The model that the person has used to understand his or her beliefs can be elicited fairly early in this exploratory process. Some beliefs may be easily understandable: a voice heard may be that of someone who tormented or abused the person in earlier years. Others are less understandable: the person's body is inhabited by aliens. Whatever the belief, eliciting and understanding it is central to assisting the person in dealing with it and its possible consequences effectively. Romme and Escher (1989) described the individual explanations—beliefs about their voices—that a group of voice hearers had developed for their experiences, and we have found these groups of explanations accord with those proposed by people with delusions. These are listed under the headings that the authors used to classify them and some (in italics) that we have added in Table 9.1.

Use of Guided Discovery to Understand Antecedents of Delusional Beliefs

Understanding the initial events that led to the development of delusional beliefs is of great importance. This is more straightforward in cases where onset was abrupt. It is more difficult when there was a very gradual development of the symptoms. In the latter cases, the relevant events may have occurred over a number of months or years, with no precisely determinable moment of onset. However, most people will eventually point to events or circumstances that they think were important. At times, you will have to elicit these from family members or friends, or examine old medical records. They may or may not have caused the psychosis, but the significance of these events to future management can be incalculable by assisting you in understanding how and

---

TABLE 9.1. Individual Explanations of Experiences

- Psychodynamic: "they are representations of trauma that has been repressed"
- Jungian: "impulses from the unconscious speaking"
- Mystical: "part of a mind expansion"
- *Spiritual: derived from God or the devil*
- Parapsychological: "caused by a special gift or sensitivity, expanded consciousness, aliens, witchcraft, astrological forces"
- Medical: "due to a chemical imbalance, schizophrenia"
- *Technological explanations: "satellites, electromagnetism, silicon chips, etc."*

Note. Developed from Romme and Escher (1989).

why the beliefs developed. Clients will regularly describe life events whose impact has clearly been severe and distressing, such as a divorce, the death of a spouse, witnessing a murder or severe assault, being assaulted or sexually abused themselves, a serious accident, or being unfairly accused of a crime or misdemeanor that led to job loss or relationship damage. In other cases, the event may seem inconsequential until the significance to the individual becomes clear.

For still others, there may be many minor stresses—such as leaving home for college or changing one's work shift from day to night—to which the person proved particularly vulnerable. Even more subtly, they may have had reasons in the past to be suspicious of others' intentions for example, when they have been bullied—and then an event suddenly "confirms" their belief. Or, they may be seeking positive reassurance and then falsely read what they are hoping to see into developing events, resulting in shock or disappointment.

The Picture of the Prodromal Period: Events, Beliefs, Images

With some people, the onset of their illness is clearly etched on their mind, while others find it difficult, seem to be unable, or may not want to remember. When the events are clearly remembered and do not cause undue distress, a detailed description can be taken. In other cases, you will need forms of prompting or will have to have the information supplemented from other sources. When the person seems not to want to remember, it's worth checking out whether this is the case:

> "Is it too uncomfortable to remember? . . . Maybe we can come back to it later, when you are ready."

While the hesitation may reflect discomfort or painful memories, clients may also be paranoid, suspicious of your motives, or just embarrassed in cases where they have some insight and think they will appear foolish.

Whenever a direct approach to unearthing relevant information seems appropriate, ask whichever of the following questions seems a reasonable starting point:

> "When did your problems begin?"
>
> "When did you first think that . . . ?"
>
> "When did you last feel well?"
>
> "When did you first see a doctor about these problems?"
>
> "When did you first see a psychiatrist [or psychologist, nurse, or counselor] about these problems?"
>
> "When were you first hospitalized?"

Sometimes a series of events will be described, perhaps even going back into childhood, and while these may not be psychotic experiences, they will be important in developing a formulation.

> Leonard had grown up as an only child on a farm and had been quite isolated from other children outside school. Unfortunately, at school he had been bullied repeat-

edly and had a very unhappy childhood. On leaving school, he worked on the farm for a few years before joining the army. Within a few weeks bullying began again, and on this occasion he reacted, hit an officer, and was confined to a small cell in the army camp. Within a day he had developed a psychotic illness with agitation, paranoid beliefs, and hallucinations.

The client might choose to describe transient experiences that seem linked in some way to the person prior to the initial psychotic episode, or he or she may recognize specifically distressing or confusing events. Try to establish when the first positive and even negative symptoms occurred in order to define the initial experience thoroughly.

However, even such questions as the foregoing may not provide much useful information, particularly when onset has been gradual. An assessment session focusing on an initial discussion or recap of the personal history will often help. As you review the circumstances relating to birth, childhood, adolescence, schooling, and subsequent years, either the person begins to describe the initial experience or it becomes apparent that he or she has jumped forward to a period after its onset. There are times (especially when a person has been institutionalized for years) when accessing this information is very difficult, but in the end, with prompts from other sources and the development of a therapeutic relationship, someone—whether it be a nurse, or even a nursing or medical student innocently trying to get a psychiatric history—usually encounters this information.

When it is clear that the time of onset has been bypassed in the personal history, try backtracking:

"So, you were just saying that you had been put in the hospital. How did that happen?"

"Who was there? Were your parents present? Did you get there in an ambulance? Was that from your home?"

"So, what were you doing when the ambulance came? Had you seen a doctor? Do remember what he or she said?"

"Do you remember how you were feeling? Do you remember what you'd been doing? Had you had any fights or disagreements with anyone?"

It may be necessary to ask many questions, and this certainly needs to be done sensitively. Repeated questioning should be used with caution, and you will find that some people are better able to cope with such a structured approach when closed questions (answered with a "yes" or "no") are used more frequently than open questions.

THERAPIST: How are you feeling today?

PHILIP: All right.

THERAPIST: Any worries or problems?

PHILIP: No.

THERAPIST: Do you mind if I ask you a few questions?

PHILIP: OK.

THERAPIST: I gather you checked into the hospital because of a few problems at home . . . with the neighbors?

PHILIP: Yes.

THERAPIST: Were they upsetting you in some way?

PHILIP: Yes, they were listening to me through the walls.

THERAPIST: Oh . . . How long do you think they've been doing that?

PHILIP: Since last Christmas.

THERAPIST: Did something happen, then—an argument or something?

PHILIP: (*Pause*) I don't want to talk about it.

THERAPIST: OK. How are you getting on here in the ward? Have you got enough to do? [Or: Are you having any visitors? What's the food like? Are you watching this program on TV? How's your basketball/baseball/football team doing? Etc.]

As in the example, you may need to shift the focus to more general and nonspecific discussion and then return later to more closed questions when the person is relaxed and able to supply information. If the client becomes unduly agitated, this process should also be followed.

As details emerge of the events that were relevant, it is possible to create a picture—almost a "witness statement"—showing what happened. Details should include:

"Where were you?"

"Who were you with?"

"What happened?"

"How did it happen?"

"What did you say? What did they say?"

"How long did it last?"

"And then what happened?"

Such discussion enables you to construct a clear, logical, and chronological account. You may at times need to draw the person back to the time sequence or sometimes work in chunks of the narrative until you have the sequence of words and actions in correct order. As far as possible, allowing the person's account to flow naturally is better than interrupting, but whenever irrelevant topics are being introduced or repetition is occurring, you may need to reroute the discussion to maximize clarity and tie up loose ends.

This process involves identifying significant life events and occurrences. Although on the surface the account of the beginning of a psychotic illness may not seem to involve dramatically stressful events, it is worth repeating that often they may be most significant ones in the etiology of the condition. The reasons for their significance may already be obvious from the personal history and an understanding of the person's life circumstances, or they may emerge only later after the links between thoughts, feelings, and beliefs are filled in.

While this is an extension of the assessment process, it is also often therapeutic. It may even be the first time that the person has been able to discuss the whole sequence of events and therefore begin to assess their meaning and consequences. When such was attempted previously, the person may have been too psychotic or thought-disordered or just unable or unwilling to trust the person trying to elicit that information. For many it will be the first time for quite a long time for these matters to be discussed therapeutically, and such an undertaking is often greatly appreciated.

When the client's story appears to be complete, one can start to examine it. Generally speaking, proceeding to therapeutic intervention before completing the client's story (i.e., without at least a good framework of events) can be risky. The therapist risks jumping to conclusions about matters that may seem wholly delusional but are actually factually supported. Such a misstep can seriously, even fatally, harm your relationship and ability to work with the person.

How do you determine when the client's story is complete enough? Often the person will let you know that he or she has told you all that is relevant. Alternatively, the picture that emerges must appear to be a coherent and reasonably complete explanation—which will become more apparent when a formulation is drawn up.

Finding Connections between Activating Events, Beliefs, and Consequences

As significant events unfold, so often do the thoughts about them, such as:

"I thought I was going to die."

"I imagined being locked up forever."

And this type of exposition needs to be encouraged by simple prompting, for example:

"Why did you think that?"

"Did you wonder what was going to happen?"

There may be a temptation to direct attention toward feelings, such as by asking "How did that make you feel?," which we tend to resist (although it's often reasonable to open discussions by asking "How are you feeling today?"). There may be circumstances in which eliciting feelings can be rapport-enhancing (see Chapter 4 on the therapeutic relationship) or can be necessary to connect with thoughts but generally not at this juncture, where exploration of thoughts about events is the goal.

At this stage, thoughts may be presented as facts, for example:

"That was when the neighbors started bugging my phone."

If you think that the person is well engaged, it may be worth gently reframing:

"So, that was when it first occurred to you that the neighbors had started bugging your phone?"

If in doubt, however, it's perfectly acceptable to leave the statement as it stands at this point in proceedings. As the key beliefs emerge, so they can be explored individually to understand how they developed.

The ABC framework used in other areas of cognitive therapy may be helpful in clarifying the relationship between events and beliefs (see Figure 9.1). It can be used to distinguish between activating events, beliefs, and consequences, as these frequently become confused, with people jumping from *A*'s to *C*'s without considering the intermediary belief. Examining each part of the sequence can clarify it and allow the person to begin to question assumptions (Chadwick et al., 1996).

At this stage, other negative thoughts may be emerging, and these affect the individual similarly to other conditions (such as depression), among which are:

- Personalization ("taking things personally")
- Selective abstraction ("getting things out of context")
- Arbitrary inference ("jumping to conclusions")
- Minimizing
- Maximizing ("making mountains out of molehills")
- Overgeneralization
- Dichotomous reasoning ("all-or-nothing thinking")

Such cognitive errors are central to understanding delusional beliefs. While it is perfectly normal to center one's attention on oneself, it can be easy to take things too personally, especially when there is no external feedback (e.g., from friends or family, who are available or with whom there is a trusting relationship). This can also occur when the person suffers from sensory impairment (e.g., deafness or blindness) that need not be complete but that interferes with functioning sufficiently to affect clarity of communication and confidence.

Such impairments can mean that events that are inconsequential are made to *seem* consequential. Someone in the street is heard to say "That's a rip-off" and the person mistakenly thinks it refers to him- or herself—"That means I'm a rip-off" (in other words, useless). The context may quickly be forgotten. For example, a procession of large black cars coming slowly down the road may be taken to mean that "It is the Mafia being sent to get me" when in reality it is a funeral procession. A bus doesn't come—"That means that the police have intercepted it because they saw I was waiting for it, so

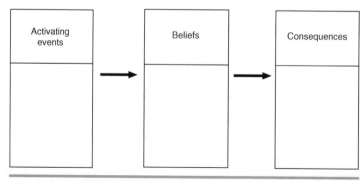

FIGURE 9.1. ABC model.

TABLE 9.2. **Understanding Experiences**

- Let the person lead.
- Explore the person's models of his or her mental health problems first.
- Normalize but don't minimize.
- Use the vulnerability–stress model to explain illness.
  - Identify vulnerabilities: family history, birth difficulties, "sensitive personality,", brain injury.
  - Identify stressors (possibly describe evidence): work, school, college, sexual relationships, and in drug or alcohol abuse.

that I will not go and expose them." Voices say "You are hopeless"—"and the fact that I forgot to get cereal for my son for breakfast tomorrow confirms that," whereas the person actually looks after his or her home and son very well (this being a case of minimizing the good and maximizing the bad, or rather a minor mistake). "Everybody on TV is talking about me" is an overgeneralization that lends itself to investigation and debate. Dichotomous reasoning ("all-or-nothing" thinking) may reinforce delusional conviction in certain circumstances through such beliefs as "all people with large noses, such as me, are ugly and will be shunned by other people." In seeking to normalize the client's misperceptions of him- or herself, use the suggestions presented in Table 9.2.

Which Belief Should Be Discussed First?

If there is a choice, it probably is worth starting gently, discussing less firmly held beliefs first and then building up to exploration of those that are more central. But in practice most people are quite clear about what most concerns them and it is these areas that will have emerged during assessment and that, gently, may be broached. If the topic causes distress or even undue animation or agitation, it may be worth discussing whether the person wants to continue along these lines "today" or rather talk about something else for the remainder of the session. Generally, letting the client lead and collaboratively set the agenda for action is most appropriate.

Discussing and Debating Delusions

It is best to proceed by exploring the content of the delusion being considered fully, drawing from the information assembled about its development (see Table 9.3). In doing this, establish with the client the nature of evidence *for* the delusion—that is, what-

TABLE 9.3. **Discussing Delusions**

- Establish engagement.
- Trace the origins of the delusion.
- Build a picture of the prodromal period.
- Identify *significant* life events and circumstances.
- Identify relevant perceptions (e.g., tingling, fuzziness) and thoughts (e.g., suicidal, violent).
- Review negative thoughts and dysfunctional assumptions, especially taking things personally and getting things out of context.

ever is used to support the belief—supplement that evidence with relevant information of your own, if available. For example, there may be relevant information from world events occurring at the time of onset of the belief that might seem to suggest delusional interpretations, certainly paranoid or government-based ones. For example, client might believe that the government is spying on him or her and then a local newspaper reports that the customs service has been monitoring local shops for contraband goods. It would be perfectly acceptable for the therapist to initiate a discussion, for example, of the increasing use of surveillance via video cameras or closed circuit TV, thereby intruding unduly into people's privacy.

We have never known frank discussion such as this to worsen symptoms by being incorporated into the person's delusions or delusional system, or reinforcing his or her fears. On the contrary, it enhances the therapist–client relationship by taking the belief seriously—at face value—and trying to understand it through the use of appropriate supporting evidence. It also tends to improve the client's ability and desire to be self-critical by focusing the discussion on related circumstances. It sometimes feels uncomfortable providing information that fits in with a strong and apparently delusional belief, but if such information exists there are major advantages in bringing it up at this point. If the information surfaces belatedly, the client may well think you have deceived him or her, or not acted evenhandedly.

Often subsequent *confirmatory* evidence emerges by chance to reinforce beliefs. Paranoia in particular can be reinforced by other people's attitudes. If they become adverse or distant because of negativity or nonresponsiveness from the client, his or her paranoid is further reinforced. This can also occur in relation to the involvement of mental health services, psychiatrists, hospitalization or medication—especially if these services are against the person's wishes—as any such actions can readily be perceived in a paranoid way. Other delusions can also receive reinforcement: for example, hypochondriacal beliefs can lead to increased symptoms of anxiety with corresponding physical symptoms and spiritual beliefs may be reinforced by statements in books (such as religious books) or by media developments that may be open to a number of interpretations. Increased paranoia can also result from the side effects of medication—for example, tremors or dystonic reactions (involuntary muscular movements) that may seem like others controlling them—or sexual side effects (e.g., impaired erection and ejaculation) or the effects by medication on prolactin (a body hormone), causing breast enlargement or the secretion of breast milk, which can inspire delusions about gender change or becoming pregnant.

Be thorough and consistent, follow through on any anomalies arising between what is said and what was reported to have occurred. Exploring *disconfirmatory* evidence needs to be done very sensitively and Socratically, using guided discovery as the predominant approach. Eliciting evidence from the client is far more persuasive than presenting it to him or her yourself. "Challenging" is probably not the best way to describe this approach, since discussion that is too assertive can be intimidating. Even a hint of conflict can undo much successful work, leading the person into psychological reactance; that is, if they feel driven into a corner, they begin to defend at all costs and become much less open to discussing alternative ways of considering their experiences and beliefs. Pointing out anomalies to the person may be necessary, but in our experience it is a much less successful approach than letting the person identify anomalies firsthand.

Sometimes bringing in others who are liked or respected by the person can help—

but done in a gentle way as far as possible with their consent. These significant others need not be present for you to discuss their opinions with the person, although their involvement in interviews *can* be helpful. Asking the client to check out beliefs with close friends and family may be a useful way of exploring beliefs in a nonconfrontational manner, as in, for example:

"What does your sister think about this?"

"Why do you think your husband thinks that?"

Sometimes the introduction of a new viewpoint clarifies beliefs, as other factors of importance in explaining the beliefs emerge—to the extent that sometimes a seemingly delusional belief turns out to have an element of truth in it, or at least to be understandable. At the same time, being able to view the beliefs from another's perspective can increase the person's critical evaluation of the belief. The therapist might ask:

"If someone said that [i.e., what you just said] to *you*, how would *you* respond?"

Generation of Alternative Explanations and Further Research to Explore Them

Introducing the idea that there may be an alternative interpretation of the events or perceptions that have apparently been delusionally interpreted needs great care, as it is easy for the client to jump to the conclusion that

"You don't believe me either—you're all the same!"

If the person can be led to consider alternative possibilities with minimal prompting, this is much preferable—and sometimes nonverbal guidance, a frown or puzzled look from the therapist, may be appropriate with a gentle prompt if one is needed. So often the development of the formulation leads to the person beginning to question, albeit silently, beliefs which previously he or she took as self-evident.

But if no progress is being made through the client's looking for alternatives, it may be safe to prompt:

"Any other possible explanations for what happened?"

Gently prompting about specific possibilities may be in order, although again if the person can present without prompting that is certainly better:

"What about . . . ? Do you think just possibly . . . ?"

How far to explore alternatives depends on how open the person is to doing so. If he or she seems quite guarded and resistant, it may be appropriate to explore development of the delusion but move to methods of dealing with persistent delusions, described later in this chapter, relatively quickly—although it is very important to be sure that the beliefs have been sufficiently explored first.

Normalizing information, described previously (in Chapter 8), can be usefully and nonthreateningly introduced and may assist where relevant, for example about suggestibility—which is associated with feeling anxious and confused—and "brainwashing." Finding meaning can be enormously reassuring and anxiety-reducing, but does not necessarily suggest that the meaning found is the correct explanation. Also, understanding automatic thoughts and anxiety symptoms can help in cases where these appear to have been misconstrued.

Generation of Testable Hypotheses

Testing beliefs can assist in clarifying them, and, in cases where they are not strongly held, in developing alternative ways of looking at events and situations. Diaries are useful in identifying when beliefs occur and what they are precisely about. However, any tasks that are set as goals need to be simple and worthwhile from the standpoint of the person asked to accomplish the task—otherwise, they will not be successful. It may be necessary—indeed the person may want—to set up a specific test (e.g., if they believe that they can foretell the future, that a certain agreed-upon thing will happen at a set date or time). Such tests may sow doubt when the prediction does not occur, however, usually a reason is given that leaves the belief as unshakeable as before.

Hypothetical contradiction—which involves asking the person whether there are *any* circumstances in which they might reverse their belief—has also been suggested as a way of proceeding. This can seem contrived and, while useful possibly in assessing the degree of delusional conviction, may have limitations as a therapeutic technique, as it potentially impairs engagement. The client's typical attitude is:

"You don't believe me, do you? I've told you there is no way I could be wrong!"

Use of Research and Homework to Explore the Person's Explanations of Specific Events or Beliefs

Exploration or investigation of evidence for beliefs can be considered. Many people with schizophrenia have a marked aversion to the term "homework," negatively associating it with school days, so we tend to avoid it. Any theoretical proposition may invite further investigation, however; for example:

"Can satellites influence people's movements?"

"How can we find out about this?"

"Do you know much about satellites?"

"How can we find out more?"

"We could search the library or Internet. We could write to somebody about it, but we'd need to find out who might know."

The use of relevant self-help material or searching in encyclopedias or the Internet may be of value. But don't expect the client to do this. Our experience is that clients will usually look at material you bring in and appreciate the effort you have made but normally not search for much themselves. When exceptionally they do offer to do so and follow it up, this can be a major development in therapy. But you may find that, as you take the client's belief more and more seriously and investigate it further and further, he or she tends to lose interest in it! What emerges, however, is an accessibility to work with key personal issues, and often behavior based on or influenced by the delusional beliefs begins to change.

People with multiple symptoms (e.g., voices and thought disorder) may switch to different symptoms when progress seems to be occurring in one area. Those with fixed monodelusional states and systematized delusions can simply become frustrated, and further debate becomes counterproductive. However, this need not be a reason for undue concern, as, on many occasions, you've now sown the seed and can await development (see Table 9.4).

PERSISTENT DELUSIONS

When you find yourself going around in circles or following ever extending delusional beliefs or the person is getting annoyed, it's sensible to stand back and take stock. Has the person said something significant about his or her life that may seem quite unrelated to the delusional beliefs but is of importance in its own right? If so, pursue it, if they are agreeable—it is perfectly reasonable to stop trying to reason with clients about their delusions and move to topics of self-evident importance. (While this may seem obvious, sometimes therapists can become so engrossed in working on specific delusions, they can fail to notice important emerging themes that seem, at best, tenuously related but of considerable importance in their own right).

If such themes are not emerging, what problems are prominent for this person? What goals does he or she have? How can we help the client achieve the goals despite the beliefs and their consequences?

Ask yourself: What purpose does the belief seem to serve? The possibilities are numerous:

- Gives a purpose to life (e.g., searching for "my real" father).
- Improves self-esteem or protects against despair.
- Affects personal relationships, for example, with parents.

TABLE 9.4. Debating Delusions

- Explore the content of the delusion.
- Establish the nature of the evidence for the delusion.
- Discuss subsequent *confirmatory* evidence, including the side effects of medication (e.g., dystonia)
- Be thorough and follow through on any anomalies that arise: for example, be the basset hound, *not* the terrier, and Colombo, *not* "Dirty Harry"
- Consider, discussing significant others' opinions: for example, "Why do you think they think that?"
- Elicit alternatives: "Any other possibilities?" or "If someone said that to you, how would you respond?"
- Gently prompt: "What about . . . ? Do you think just possibly . . . ?
- Explore and investigate (not as "homework") any theoretical proposition—but don't expect the client to do it.
- Sew seeds and remain observant for possible developments.

- Prevents facing the anxieties associated with the need to work, make friends, and so forth.
- Protects against a greater underlying fear, for example, that I'm useless, or I have cancer.
- Explains anomalous or confusing situations—for example, fatigue from depression must be due to poisoning by neighbors.
- Provides something to talk about—or at least this element contributes to the overall picture.

More often than not, there is an element of truth in beliefs. You should not be reluctant to admit that to the client. Occasionally the situation may arise where you can't see *anything wrong* with a particular belief. You will need to be clear whether others do and if so why. Otherwise as further information becomes available, you may be in a difficult situation, having to backtrack with the client and losing credibility. If you cannot progress or at least are now going to stop trying to work directly with the belief, identify what issues there are: "Do we need to help you cope with it and the possible consequences?" Suggest practical measures that might help—for example, "If you are worried about being assaulted, why not take a siren with you? Or get physically fit."

Following the Logic of the Belief (Inference Chaining)

For many people in whom beliefs seem to be fixed and resistant to any form of rational response, it is still possible to do very useful work by using some form of inference chaining. For example:

> "If others agreed with you about your belief that [*state belief*], what would it mean to you? How would it affect you?"

This is a very effective and nonthreatening way to find out what is important about the belief. With grandiose beliefs, people will frequently talk about issues that have to do with self-esteem—for example, "I'll be respected." Other needs invite other responses—often difficult to predict from the assessment and even from the formulation, for example, "I'd feel happier," "I'd have a girlfriend," or "I wouldn't be lonely." Having identified a general need, it may pay to get more specific for example, "But whom do you particularly want to be respected by?" Often such inference chaining provides specific information about circumstances that can be worked with. The unmet need may be related to a particular, especially family, relationship:

> CLIENT: My father would show me some respect.
>
> THERAPIST: Well, if this is related to respect from your father, is it OK for us to talk about this a bit more? Why do you think there are these differences between you and your father?

Working directly with the family and the support of the client in understanding his or her difficulties can begin to lead to changes in the relationship—or sometimes just the perception of it. The issue about loneliness or having a girlfriend, once raised by the client in this context, can often allow exploration and motivation to change in an area that has been fraught with difficulties and often previously resisted by the person. This may even be where change is obviously required and has previously been identified as a key area—discussing it by approaching it through the delusional system can open it up. For example:

> "I can't help you with your claim to be Eminem's spiritual companion, but we might be able to help you with the loneliness you are feeling."

There is certainly a time to stop trying to reason directly with delusional beliefs. Indeed after full assessment, exploration, and work on seeking alternative explanations, taking the focus off the beliefs may be necessary for progress to be made. Trying for too long and too hard is much more of a problem than changing tack too early—assuming that you have developed a good relationship with the client.

Work can then focus on problem solving and developing short-term (in terms of days and weeks) and long-term (months and years) goals for the future. It may well be that specific incidents from the person's past or specific current concerns need work in much the same way that management of depression and anxiety does. Indeed, it may be that social phobia, obsessional symptoms, and social problems (e.g., housing) take precedence for your attention. It may seem as though you are avoiding the key issues—that is, the delusional beliefs or voices—but in practice and in fact the key issues are the ones you are now dealing with: those of everyday living. It is just that the delusional beliefs and voices have often prevented the person from confronting them before. Now, having established a therapeutic relationship and developed a formulation, the person may not be able to look at his or her beliefs differently—or at least tell you that this is happening—but in time this may be possible. Direct confrontation just sets up a reaction that entrenches the beliefs rather than permitting the client to slowly move on. The client may start to collaborate with you over medication or other forms of care—gently, unobtrusively, but definitely. Others, for example, caregivers—formal and informal—will start to give positive feedback. The client's mood begins to improve and activity gradually develops, but it can take quite a lot of time—often months—before this picture becomes obvious and years before goals are achieved (see Table 9.5).

WORK WITH SCHEMAS

Finally, there can be no dispute that people organize what they perceive into categories that allow them to develop some understanding of their perceptions, described as schemas. It is also clear that sometimes these ways of understanding the world or parts of it can be distorted and distressing. Beck and colleagues have described ways in which personality can be understood, and, with it, certain key beliefs may be delineated, for example, "I am unlovable." Work on these underlying beliefs forms an important part of work with emotional and personality disorders. These beliefs are self-evidently undesirable. However, it is unclear whether working with such beliefs in psychosis is useful or indeed possible, and the research evidence is inconclusive. People rarely make such universal statements as "I am unlovable" but may accede to them when presented the opportunity—arguably, the therapeutic aim may become demolishing the "straw doll" that has been constructed. By this point, however, the overwhelming feeling of being, for example, universally unlovable, has been interpreted

TABLE 9.5. **Resistant Delusions**

- If becoming agitated or hostile, stop and get help.
- If not, agree to differ, stand back, and:
  —Review key issues and concerns that have emerged
  —Consider inference chaining
    o Factual implications: "If you have a silicon chip in your brain, doesn't it need electricity to work?"
    o Emotional underpinning, concerns, or consequences of beliefs: "OK, I do have some problems with this . . . but if other people did accept what you are saying, what difference would that make to you,' what would distress you most about it,' what could you do about it,' and why would it be so important?"
    o Follow through to specific changes in relationships, etc: "I'd be respected." "By whom in particular?" "My husband and daughter."
    o Then deal with the emerging issue: "Although I may not be able to accept that you're a member of the royal family, I may be able to help you work things out with your husband."
    o Explain procedures: "If the police come to arrest you, ring this number [solicitor] and contact us."
    o Adapt inference chain to the content of the delusion; proceed very sensitively, don't be crass: for example, not "If you were the richest man in the world, what difference would that make to you?" but instead "Of course, if you were the richest man in the world, you could buy just about anything, but what would be the most important difference to your life?"

and taken root. With psychotic people in particular but also with others, this can be emotionally overwhelming or at least seriously damaging to engagement, even if acknowledged by the person as a reflection of what he or she believes to be true.

Changes in schemas may well occur through behavior or experiences that validate the person (e.g., the experience of being loved). It is less clear that debate about the thoughts does this. Downward-arrow techniques, questioning methods that drill down to and then focus on "hot cognitions"—emotionally powerful thoughts—may be too unsettling for people with psychosis and may have negative effects. It is possible that such may be tolerated by some, but whether they can shift delusional ideas or voices is uncertain. It may be therapeutic to elicit negative comments that may come straight from the content of delusions or voices, but this is so that the comments can be promptly examined and discussed; for example:

CLIENT: My voices say "You're useless."

THERAPIST: Do you believe that?

CLIENT: Yes. [The person will often say this tentatively or deny that he or she is wholly useless.]

THERAPIST: Can we look at why you believe that? [You can then develop a "balance sheet" and weigh the reasons for and against this proposal.]

A further example:

CLIENT: The neighbors are following me. [You could look at evidence for believing this or possible reasons for their actions—or explore both alternatives at different times.]

THERAPIST: Why do you think they would want to do that?

CLIENT: Because they think I'm bad (or that I've done something bad).

THERAPIST: Could we discuss why you believe that? [Use a similar "weighing" process.]

Understanding schemas may be useful, but direct work on them needs to be considered carefully and probably is best done with minimal arousal of distress. As with all areas, if the person is starting to get distressed, it is probably best to take a different direction after lessening the person's distress level.

SPECIFIC TYPES OF DELUSIONS

Although the principles and practices described above apply to all work with delusions, there are some differences in terms of emphasis with different delusional content, and so the following delusional types will be mentioned briefly.

Grandiose Delusions

Grandiose delusions can take the form of beliefs that the person has special powers, for example, that he or she can:

- Foretell the future
- Read people's thoughts
- Control others' actions
- Heal others
- Invent

Alternatively, the person may believe him- or herself to be a special person, sometimes a historical one, or to be an offspring of or to be in communication with such a figure. For example:

- Spiritual—God, devil, angel Gabriel, prophet
- Royal—King, Queen, Princess, Emperor (Diana, Napoleon)
- Political—President or Prime Minister of their home country or a distant country
- Scientist
- Doctor, especially a psychiatrist
- Artist

There is some emerging evidence that such beliefs may be related to issues of self-esteem (as has long been suspected) and so any attempt at undermining the belief should be resisted, although collaborative exploration remains perfectly appropriate. However with some people with recurrent grandiose episodes (or mania), the underlying belief may be more related to "being special," which in moderation is a positive attribute but in some people seems to go out of control to being "the most special person." Normalization of the belief that it is a normal human characteristic to believe you are special—especially if buoyed by some success can be therapeutic—but this needs to be tested out with others. With the few exceptions who receive external validation (e.g., winning a Nobel Prize), most of us become aware that we may be special but do not lose control of this. When control is lost, a damaging cascade of beliefs may result:

> "Because I am so special, normal rules do not apply to me. I can spend as much money as I like, drive my car as fast as I want, and everybody will be attracted to me and want to hear what I say."

Criticism and attempts to control errant behavior are dismissed as being because "these fools do not recognize me" (occasionally accompanied by the thought that, as Christ said, "a prophet is not recognized in his own country"), and any limitations placed on such persons only increase their attempts to act on their grandiose delusions.

The impact of beliefs may also be negative through the stigmatization that can occur when such grandiose notions are communicated to others—especially strangers. It may be that the first issue to be dealt with is how to adjust self-presentation to minimize outright rejection. Reasoning rarely displaces grandiose beliefs, but inference chaining and other ways of managing resistant delusions can be successful in working with underlying issues. Such beliefs shift slowly, and there is no evidence yet that work with grandiosity has negative effects—the contrary seems to be the case, as such beliefs can seriously isolate the person from others and paradoxically lead to distress from rejection. Cognitive therapy can often enable the person to reintegrate with others through behavior change, with beliefs becoming increasingly less intrusive and obsessive.

Paranoid Delusions

Paranoia is one of the commonest symptoms of schizophrenia. It usually has a focus on a person, group of people, or organization but may generalize as far as to involve everyone except the person him- or herself, for example:

- Police
- Government, whether foreign or domestic
- Secret agencies, for example, FBI and CIA
- Drug dealers, the Mafia
- Neighbors
- Family
- Mental health workers
- Strangers, especially suspicious-looking ones
- "Anybody"

It can present associated with trauma, where the paranoia may be very specifically against individuals responsible for assaults or abuse upon the person. It may be an effect of drug-precipitated illness or consequent to the development of other delusional beliefs, for example, grandiose ones ("they are after my invention"). It may be manifest as an oversensitivity associated with delusions of reference and thought broadcasting (sensitivity psychosis). In the first group, the paranoia may be associated with a belief that the person deserves punishment (described as "bad me" by Chadwick and colleagues [1996]). The second group sees themselves as undeserving "poor me," while the last group seems to take a middle position in which they seem persuadable to either viewpoint.

A major goal of therapy is to reduce overgeneralization. This means asking the person to be specific, for example:

"Who specifically and when did that person or organization say or do something against you?"

"Why should they do that?"

Examine exactly what has seemed to be happening—why that particular person or group and what their motives might be. It is well worth going out for a walk with the person or looking out of a window and asking the person about specific people as they pass:

"Are they part of the plot?"

"How did you decide that?"

"Was it something they did?"

"Or something they wore or a way they looked?"

Such questions assist the person in developing a critical position that they can then use themselves when they are outdoors. Particularly important is that it can lead to an acceptance that not everybody is against them—that there are probable exceptions.

Examining the reasons why the person believes organizations—for example, the government or police—are tracking him or her can also be therapeutic, representing an attempt to begin to depersonalizing his or her belief system.

"Why should they follow you?"

"How many men do you think it takes? How much would that cost?"

"What could you have done that warrants that?"

"Have you complained against the organization?"

"Do you think this is just being done to you or lots of other people?"

Such reasoning approaches can be quite successful, especially within the context of a good therapeutic relationship, although again instances may develop where techniques for persistent delusions need to be used. Protective measures against the person's fears may be discussed. Some of these may include increasing security (such as carrying a personal alarm, increasing locks on doors), and it is not clear whether on balance these help—that is, are perceived as supportive—or whether they reinforce the paranoid beliefs. Until clear evidence emerges about this, the person's preference should rule.

Spiritual Delusions

Distinguishing spiritual delusions from spiritual beliefs held by others can be difficult, especially when people from the person's spiritual or cultural group are not available to assist and the assessor is from a significantly different cultural background. Beliefs may also be understandable elaborations or concrete interpretations of spiritual teachings. Nevertheless, collaborative nonjudgmental exploration can clarify matters.

Spiritual beliefs about voices or attributes (e.g., of being a prophet) can be quite resilient to change because of the conviction that it is God's message or voice that is being heard or occurring. Whereas one might expect other people to hear sounds such as voices that are loud and insistent (see Chapter 10 on hallucinations), this is not necessarily to be expected if the voice comes from God or the devil. Spiritual beliefs anticipate unusual and seemingly irrational things happening, and so again standard reasoning may not be applicable.

However, it may be possible to compare the spiritual beliefs with spiritual teachings. For example, the language and condemnation of many voices contrasts with a forgiving God—although discussions about the more vengeful God of the Old Testament, if the person is knowledgeable about this, may be more difficult. (Generally the superceding of this by the New Testament may be a route to explore.) As with all symptoms, mood can determine content—and vice versa—so work on mood and self-esteem as well as the beliefs is most likely to be successful.

Some delusions with a spiritual theme will be quite resistant to direct reasoning approaches but be susceptible to inference chaining, as previously described:

"If others believed that you were a prophet, would that be important to you?"

"In what way would that make a difference?"

Usually responses will be about self-esteem or loneliness or similar themes, and the person may then allow you to address these matters directly.

Bizarre Delusions

Exactly how you treat comments that seem extreme—for example, "I have an alien inside my body"—depends on the level of engagement. It is certainly important to treat them as if they are rational and potentially understandable statements even if you have difficulty understanding how they can be. If the relationship is building well, it can be acceptable and therapeutic to introduce some verbal and nonverbal questioning—a frown—and:

"I don't quite understand that. . . . When you say alien, can you explain a bit more what you mean?—something feeling alien?"

They may then expand and explain it. It may be meant literally—or metaphorically.

A safer route, especially where it is proving difficult to elicit information, may be to say:

"That sounds frightening . . . is that how you feel?"

"Or do you feel something different? For example, angry at feeling this. . . . Or even . . . proud at its choosing you?"

"How does it affect you? Does it stop you doing anything or make you do things you don't want to do?"

"Since when?"

"How did it enter?"

"How is it nurtured?"

"Why does it stay? Can it leave if it wished to?"

"Currently what are the signs that it is there?"

"What about others' reactions? Are they aware of it? Have you told anyone? What did they say?"

Especially with bizarre delusions—of aliens, vampires, and so forth—it is worth checking out whether these relate to a song, film, or TV program, as is often the case. Sometimes doing this helps you understand what the person is describing, may make him or her feel you understand, and may also make a connection with film or TV. Either this can begin to sow doubt in the person's mind or allow you to begin to work with the belief effectively! A concrete belief arising from a very convincing film sometimes seems to be the origin of a bizarre delusion.

Check how energy is provided for the silicon chip (etc.). How was it inserted, if that was what happened? Explain the procedures for operations, if relevant—for example, the need for informed consent. Who is doing it? If unsure, it is often worth prompting with possibilities—for example, the CIA, aliens, witches, neighbors. Why should they do it? What do they have to gain? How much must it cost in time and resources? What have you done to warrant such attention?

Sometimes delusional beliefs are derived from physical symptoms of anxiety. Tingling (paresthesia) can occur with hyperventilation, as can giddiness and aches and pains. When the person doesn't understand, as many people don't, that these can be anxiety-related, he or she will look for another explanation. Perhaps it is a physical illness—cancer or a "nerve problem"—and depending on the person's own personal experience of such disorders, relate it to him or her. So, the "nerve problem" may be multiple sclerosis or dementia or a brain tumor. Understanding anxiety can be very important in providing an alternative explanation and general anxiety management techniques, including the use of person information leaflets, useful in again sowing doubt where previously certainty existed.

Many beliefs do shift, especially when they are part of a constellation of symptoms, for example, accompanied by voices or other delusions (particularly in sensitivity and drug-related disorders). Some, especially monosymptomatic psychoses (as in anxiety psychosis), do not shift with these reasoning techniques alone.

Hypochondriacal Beliefs

Hypochondriacal beliefs can arise in several forms. Most common are false convictions that:

- Certain parts of the body are definitely (contrary to others' opinions) misshapen or ugly.
- He or she has a specific physical illness.

- Part of the body is not functioning.
- The person experiences chronic pain.
- He or she emits a foul odor from the skin, mouth, rectum, or (for women) vagina.
- There is an infestation of insects on or in the skin.
- There is an internal parasite.

Interventions need to be administered as part of a broad comprehensive package of care addressing social needs and issues having to do with relationships. Many people presenting with hypochondriacal disorders are isolated and may require support in developing social networks, but may be very resistant to doing so.

Cognitive-behavioral techniques used for hypochondriacal beliefs, which are not considered to be delusional, may be appropriate and should not be overlooked with this group. Their use with these more bizarre and entrenched symptoms involves a similar structured and collaborative approach. People with monosymptomatic hypochondriacal psychosis (i.e., single fixed beliefs) are notoriously difficult to engage and react vehemently if the suggestion is made—or they interpret it as being made—that they are "imagining" their somatic symptom. Suggestions about stress are likewise dismissed, so that a method of intervention that provides minimal prompts is indicated, even though it may seem slow. Many of this group will resist attending clinics to see psychiatrists or psychologists but may be prepared to be seen in community settings, for example, health centers or family doctor's surgeries, or even in their homes. Introduction by an intermediary (e.g., the family doctor or practice nurse) may also be helpful. A Socratic approach needs to be used that involves gentle questioning and exploration to draw on the person's own beliefs and ideas about their problems without preconceptions. In this circumstance, saying something such as the following may be best:

> "I've just come because your doctor asked me to. It may be a complete waste of both our time, but if you can just explain what the problem is, I can go and talk with him about it."

Therapy focuses on understanding concerns, for example, of infestation or bodily change, and by a process of guided discovery examines the development of these concerns, the circumstances in which the person found him- or herself, any relevant life stresses, and particularly the specific sensations that have been interpreted as being caused by the infestation or bodily change. Alternative explanations are developed, ideally through suggestions by the person him- or herself, and specific reasons for such sensations—especially as symptoms of anxiety—are explored. Direct debate, and certainly confrontation, rarely changes the belief. But gentle exploration may lead to engagement and allow a relationship to build that enables other important areas to be explored. Sometimes agreeing on tasks to explore and "reality test" the beliefs further can be effective. It may be that the techniques used successfully in treatment of resistant delusions described earlier can be beneficial. Following exploration and engagement, these techniques involve inference chaining the belief to understand the person better; for example:

> "I accept that you find these symptoms particularly distressing."
> "Which effect on your life is disturbing you the most?"

This may then be supplemented, if necessary, by:

"Is it the pain or discomfort?"

"Is it that you can't work to support your family or help your mother?"

"Is it that you are ashamed of what's happening?"

"Is it that it makes you isolated?"

It may then be that these individual issues can be dealt with directly. If discomfort is a factor:

"Although we don't seem to be able to get rid of your discomfort, could we look at ways of helping you cope better with it?"

Dealing with isolation would involve supported reintroduction to social networks. By initially focusing on the delusional idea and working through it, people are sometimes more prepared to accept "compromise solutions." The aim needs to be to reduce distress and disability caused by the symptoms rather than removal of the belief. The latter may later follow after the focus is taken off of it and after underlying needs are dealt with.

Olfactory Delusions

Olfactory delusions—beliefs usually that the person him- or herself smells—are particularly common and can be managed similarly to other delusional beliefs. Often the symptom is related to social anxiety and delusions of reference; that is, the person may be misinterpreting social situations in terms of personal rejection with the further explanation that it must be because he or she smells.

CASE FORMULATION AND INTERVENING WITH DELUSIONS

Gordon (*sensitivity psychosis*): The delusional beliefs that Gordon experienced were ones relating to thought broadcasting and passivity and so are dealt with in that section.

Craig (*drug-related psychosis*): Although there were many delusional beliefs, especially paranoid ones that Craig described, these were quite open to debate and discussion. They then seemed frequently to shift in prominence and not be referred to again. Their content also fluctuated, and it was other symptoms—voices, "flashbacks," and passivity—that troubled him most and needed the most work.

Gillian (*traumatic psychosis*): The focus of work was with voices but the beliefs about the voices needed to be elicited (frequently these are delusional in nature, e.g., caused by neighbors, the police, or the devil). Gillian had not explored what caused the voices in any depth but believed they were from "the tormentor." Work with these beliefs involved formulation-based links to previous events. In other words, Gillian became able to make connections between the abuse that she had experienced during in childhood and as she grew up and the beliefs and voices that she had. The belief about the "bionic arm" did not persist after hospitalization, but other fleeting delusional beliefs came and went. Simple reasoning seemed to assist, as Gillian would move on to other topics—sometimes in apparently thought-disordered fashion—as these beliefs were systematically discussed.

Paul (*anxiety psychosis*): Work with the delusional beliefs was central to therapy with Paul but was approached thorough assessment, during which a strong therapeutic relationship was developed and then comprehensive collaborative formulation. Only at this point was the evidence for and against the beliefs examined. Direct reasoning allowed an examination of the beliefs themselves and supporting evidence. Some alternatives were proposed—by Paul and the therapist—but delusional conviction did not change at this point. Preoccupation did begin to shift, and caregivers noted general nonspecific improvement. Alternative routes to further work were considered at this point: a "wait-and-see" approach that looks at practical issues, assisted by connecting delusions to specific concerns—for example, "You are concerned about the police arresting you; what can we do about that?"—and a schema-based approach.

TEN

Case Formulation and Intervening with Hallucinations

Hallucinations are conceptualized by the cognitive model as automatic thoughts that are perceived by the client as originating externally, that is, from outside of the mind. Again, a tendency to externalize combined with stressful events and circumstances precipitate these experiences. Hallucinations may be maintained by safety behaviors (e.g., avoidance) as well as dysfunctional explanations (e.g., "It is the devil speaking to me") and high levels of affect (e.g., severe distress in response to the abusive content of the voices). The client can benefit from work on reattribution, debating content, developing coping strategies, and looking at the way the hallucinations reflect beliefs that the person has about him- or herself.

AUDITORY HALLUCINATIONS

It is crucial to clarify the exact nature and impact of the hallucinatory experience: "What does it sound like? "Is it like me speaking to you—or someone shouting at you?" The modalities and triggers, as well as affective and behavioral responses, current coping approaches, linked cognitions, and attendant imagery, should all be gently explored and recorded. This will probably be the first time that the person has given a full detailed description of the experience of hearing voices. It should be confirmed with feedback and a capsule summary in order that the exact nature of the problems can be agreed upon. It is then possible to move on to construct a collaborative agenda (see Table 10.1). The person may greatly benefit at this point from hearing other voice hearers' views on their symptoms. Attendance at a Hearing Voices Network meeting or a voices group (where these exist) often helps the person to feel supported and less isolated when beginning to take back some control over these experiences.

The client's model of the experience of hearing voices should always be worked through first in a systematic and nonconfrontational manner. People usually either have no explanation—"It's just something strange"—or they have an explanation that worsens symptoms, such as "Satan is speaking to me" "The aliens are communicating

TABLE 10.1. **Working with Auditory Hallucinations**

- Clarify the exact nature of the voices and any linked symptoms.
- Work on reattribution (see Table 10.2) with the person's explanation of voice hearing, and test it out.
- Collaboratively generate other possible explanations and test these out.
- Use a voice diary to explore triggers and fluctuations in the voice hearing experience. Undertake simple environmental change if appropriate.
- Systematically work through the list of coping strategies to look for differential benefits using the diary of voices (see Appendix 5.4).
- Work to reduce linked affective exacerbators (anger, frustration, anxiety).
- Work to reduce safety behaviors if they are maintaining symptoms.
- Work using rational responding, and work with any related trauma, *or* use normalizing and exposure techniques.
- Clarify any linked schemas, and work with dysfunctional schemas that are maintaining hallucinations.
- Give booster sessions, or organize for these to be given by the case manager or mental health worker under supervision.

before abducting me," or "I have an implant in my brain that picks up and transmits radio waves." Through guided discovery and the use of additional real-world knowledge the model is elaborated and may be allocated a percentage reflecting conviction (e.g., "90% that it is God speaking"). Some other models can also be mentioned then and worked through in a similar manner (e.g., "20% due to stress"). If the voices are active during the session, then the person and therapist can try to search for any possible explanations and modes of transmission. Frequently clients have never been through this process before (see Table 10.2).

An audiotape of the voices may be attempted, especially when there is uncertainty about the voices' origins and nature. It is usually a great relief to people to realize that others cannot hear these unpleasant voices, but often for the first time they may start to question whether they are going mad or suffering from schizophrenia. This will need to be worked through in a separate session (the "Understanding Voices" leaflet in Appendix 4 may be valuable at this point). Clients can become depressed if this subject matter is not worked through optimistically but realistically. They can begin to tackle the issue of explanation by checking out with a "trusted other" (e.g., family doctor, mental health worker, ward nurse, psychiatrist, relative, or close friend) as to whether he or she can also hear the voice.

By this point the person may be curious enough to begin to use a diary of voices (see Appendix 5.4) to make a baseline record of the activity of the voice during a 7-day period. If not, a detailed recalling of the preceding week may achieve the same end. The client is encouraged to log the intensity, affective response, and any coping attempts made in relation to the different situations encountered. There is a diversity of experience with the voices, reflecting such factors as degree of stress, affect, thoughts and memories, degree of isolation and socialization, and the exact nature of the activities engaged in. During the next therapeutic session, using guided discovery these links can begin to be made and the effect of any preexisting coping strategy can be explored.

Where there is a strong emotional reaction to the voice, rational responding or behavioral approaches aimed at reducing the intensity of frustration, anger, or anxiety are often useful in reducing the distress linked to the experience.

THERAPIST: What has the voice been saying today, Allan?

ALLAN: The voice has been saying terrible things about me.

THERAPIST: Frightening and strange thoughts can happen at times of stress, but most people will blame the stress and this can reduce the upset they cause [attempt at normalizing].

ALLAN: But the voice has said and keeps saying "He is a child molester" (*angry and embarrassed*), and I would never do anything like that (*tearful, distressed*).

THERAPIST: That is just the kind of unpleasant thought that can happen if someone is very stressed out . . . It is a sign that the mind is under pressure . . . but people very rarely act on these kind of thoughts—especially when they find them so repugnant—and usually just try to shrug them off.

TABLE 10.2. **Reattribution of Auditory Hallucinations**

- Discuss the phenomena: confirm that they are not illusions or delusions of reference.
  —"Is it like someone speaking to you—like I'm doing now?"
- Explore the individuality of perception.
  —"Can anybody else hear what is said?"
  —"Not parents, friends, etc.?"
  —Check out if necessary.
    o With others, if possible.
    o Try to taperecord the voices, if they only occur when client is alone.
- Discover beliefs about origin:
  —"Why do you think others can't hear them?"
- Discuss beliefs about the origin of the voices.
  —Use techniques for delusions, if appropriate (e.g., if the answer were "It's because the FBI has a machine that generates sounds directed at individuals").
  —Explore doubts if client says, "I'm not sure how they come."
- Look for explanations:
  —"It may be schizophrenia"—discuss the meaning of this with them.
  —Cite "normalizing" alternatives: deprivation states and other stressful circumstances (e.g., bereavements, hostages, dreaming, and PTSD).
- The aim is to allow the client to consider the possibility that the voices might be his or her own thoughts.
- If they respond about the voices "They're not my thoughts, because they're somebody else," link these experiences with:
  —Dreams or "living nightmares" ("Just as you can hear others speaking when you are dreaming—in your mind—so voices may be like "dreaming awake").
  —Emotionally charged memories: events and traumas that may be "etched" on the memory and easily recalled or triggered.
  —Deprivation states.
  —"Normal" hallucinations: brink of sleep, bereavement, etc.
  —Other people's descriptions of their experiences:
    o "Hearing voices" self-help groups (if they exist in your locality) and other "voice hearers."
    o Video and written material.

ALLAN: So, I'm not a pervert, then?

THERAPIST: No ... let's try sticking with the scary thought and trying not to be afraid of it—it's a thought, not something you've done—and see what happens.

By realizing that he couldn't entirely control his thought content, particularly at times of stress, Allan relaxed much more with his unpleasant hallucination and engaged with it. He gently rationally responded to the voice that he was very happy with his girlfriend and he knew that if he became less stressed the scary thoughts would settle down.

Some clients take a very passive, disengaged approach to the voice hearing experience, often after years of distress from voices. They feel quite resigned, make no response to the voices, have given up trying any coping strategies, and avoid being angry with them but often feel very frightened and depressed by their experiences. Even this group can usually make progress by beginning to experiment with an approach that engages with the voices—that is, begins to question what the voices are saying, at least to themselves—and later even addressing the voices themselves. Having worked with his or her own coping strategies and recorded the efficacy of each approach in the diary, the client can then be introduced to the full range of possible coping strategies that individuals have used successfully in the past. Some "symptomatic" strategies that reduce distress from the voices, however, can cause such long-term difficulties as antisocial responses, social withdrawal, or using drugs or alcohol. Alternative strategies can be discussed and, if appropriate, tried one at a time to see how beneficial each might be. A list appears in Table 10.3.

Many of these potential strategies may initially make the voices slightly more prominent, depending on the individual. But it is worth systematically working with different strategies until any that are effective are found. An example of this could be coping by listening to classical music, on a walkman, developing a hobby, and then using rational responding. This can be guided through the implementation of the case formulation.

> Penny's major problem was hearing abusive voices. She had always been unassertive, and the voices had begun after she had been coerced as a teenager into a relationship with an older man. He had been physically aggressive toward her and emotionally intimidating, although she finally managed to leave him by entering a women's refuge. She quickly came to understand that the voices were her own thoughts relating back to the abuse, but she found coping strategies difficult to implement until she started to find ways to respond to the voices. This initially involved simple, much-repeated assertive statements such as "I'm not so bad," and eventually she moved on to asking the voices to "prove themselves" as she gained more confidence.

The attitude that the person takes toward the voice is the main determinant of the distress provoked by it. The person who feels him- or herself to be the powerless victim of omniscient supernatural torturing forces is usually maximally distressed and disabled. After the person has been able to state his belief (schema) about the voices (e.g., "I am powerless"), gentle approaches can be used, including:

TABLE 10.3. Examples of Coping Strategies for Auditory Hallucinations

- Behavioral control
  —For example: Taking a warm bath, going for a walk or other exercise, using a relaxation tape, using a personal tape recorder playing classical or rock music, retreating to a quiet place.
- Socialization
  —For example: friends, day centers, telling a trusted person that the voice is active and reminding yourself that nobody else can hear the voice.
- Mental health care
  —For example: using medication, calling a mental health worker.
- Symptomatic behavior (not advised!)
  —For example: getting drunk or drugged, punching a police officer, shouting at voices.
- Cognitive control
  —Distraction: for example, playing a computer game, watching TV, listening to music, doing crosswords, engaging in a hobby, doing something different from the usual routine, trying a meditation technique, prayer, a mantra, or subvocalization (for example, humming to oneself).
  —Focusing: for example, letting the voice be and relax with it.
  —Rational responding
    o Using anxiety- or anger-reducing responses to the voice content.
    o Doing something to bring the voices on (to demonstrate controllability), giving the voice a 10-minute slot at a specified time in the day, perhaps playing a cognitive therapy tape discussing voice control.
    o Using normalizing explanations, for example, explaining it as "schizophrenia playing up."
    o Combating the seemingly omniscient/omnipotent ("all-knowing, all-powerful") nature of voices. Reminding oneself that voices are not actions and need not lead to them.
    o Beginning to be assertive with the voices by developing a dialogue with them.

- Listing the evidence in relation to what the voices say.
- Working with the way voices interfere with functioning (e.g., by causing panic or avoidance).
- Using the idea of a continuum linking "normal" experience with obsessions.
- Guided imagery (e.g., reworking in the imagination responses to feared voices, situations, or individuals).
- Role play (e.g., taking the position of the voices, with the therapist responding to them or vice versa).
- Positive logging (listing positive attributes).
- Acting against the schema (initially modeled in session, e.g., demonstrating competence when voices say the person is useless).

The less confrontational techniques are used early on. Having improved the functionality of the core maladaptive schema—for example, with a change to "I can control the voice sometimes"—we can then inference chain the voice content while working with the main theme. For example:

CARL: Usually the voice says "He won't manage it . . . or . . . he will fail, as usual."

THERAPIST: If you did fail at this task, what would that mean to you?

CARL: It would be pointless to have even started.

THERAPIST: And if you never got the job started?

CARL: Then I would be a complete waste of space (*tears*).

Carl believed that his only value arose out of his achievements, but when a series of life events led him to begin to fail, his voices commenced with this theme. In this case, listing the evidence, working with the continuum, and positive logging led to a change in the underlying compensatory schema, enabling him to perceive some self-worth in relation to other personality dimensions (friendliness, loyalty, honesty, humor, etc.). The formulation-based schema work is usually helpful in working indirectly with the voice hearing experience. It is particularly effective with traumatic voices.

OTHER HALLUCINATIONS

Visual, tactile (touch), and somatic (other bodily sensations) hallucinations can occur in conjunction with schizophrenia. Visions often take the form of "flashbacks" to or associated with specific events (in traumatic psychosis) but can be bizarre ("cartoon characters" and seemingly meaningless shapes or scenes) and may be misinterpretations of, for example, "floaters" in the eyes, or related to a vivid imagination. They tend to be more fleeting than voices and so may be less distressing, but this does depend on the content and the associated affect.

Direct work with visions is similar to that with voices, involving the precise definition of the phenomena, diary logging or detailed recall to assess further, collaborative exploration of the meaning, if any, to the person, and then a formulation-based approach to understanding the visions and their associated features. Visual hallucinations are quite common following drug-induced psychoses and (as further described in Chapter 13), benefit from reattribution to those drug-induced events. The formulation can then be used to understand them and associated symptoms (see Table 10.4).

Alan presented at the age of 15 with suicidal intent, hallucinations, and "weird feelings" that seemed to be spasms, and hypersensitivity associated with panic symptoms. He had had a normal upbringing but had fallen in with a "bad crowd" at his school, got alienated from his parents, and began using "speed" (amphet-

---

TABLE 10.4. **Visual Hallucinations**

- Visions
  —Often take the form of "flashbacks" to specific events, for example, trauma- or drug-related
  —Can be bizarre and seemingly meaningless
  —May be misinterpretations
  —Tend to be fleeting and less distressing (depending on content)
- Therapy involves
  —Precise definition of the phenomena experienced
  —Use of diaries or detailed recall
  —Exploration of the meaning and associations of the vision to the person
  —Use of a formulation-based approach to understanding them

TABLE 10.5. **Somatic and Tactile Hallucinations**

- Elicit the details of their presence and frequency.
- Discuss their nature (frequently sexual or hypochondriacal).
- Discuss the mechanism:
  —"Who do you think is doing this? How are they doing it?"
  —"If you were being touched or assaulted, wouldn't someone see this happening?"
  —"Is some other method possible—rays, electricity, or magnetism? Stress?"
- Sensitively explore other explanations (e.g., sexual feelings of which the person is ashamed and may disown).
- Work on associated delusions (see Chapter 9).

amines) and ecstasy regularly. One weekend he had a particularly bad experience with drugs in which he developed visual hallucinations of aliens swirling round him and entering his body, and he became very paranoid—believing that "Chinese Triads" were after him because he had stolen some drugs. This episode led to his being admitted to the hospital and persisting symptoms subsequently. The case formulation was used to help him look back at the original episode and understand the similarities to his current symptoms—so he could begin to attribute the hallucinations "flashbacks" of the "bad trip" rather than being current and likely to threaten him now.

Somatic and tactile hallucinations are also commonly experienced phenomena in schizophrenia and can be very distressing. They can take the form of feeling as if you are being touched, especially in sexually intimate areas, and this is commonly associated with some previous sexual assault. Parts of the body (e.g., internal organs) may feel as though they are in turmoil, and beliefs may develop from these sensations (e.g., that an alien has been inserted inside oneself). Proper management, again, begins with understanding the precise nature of the phenomena: what exactly is being felt—is it discomfort, pain, touch, or movement in the body? Often these feelings relate to normal bodily functions (although sometimes embarrassing ones), which can then be discussed. Alternative explanations can be generated from an understanding of how the body works and collaboratively explored as possible reasons for the feelings experienced (see Table 10.5). Sometimes these are related to depressive delusions focused on bodily change and hypochondriasis, which require management in their own right (see Chapter 9).

CASE FORMULATION AND INTERVENING WITH HALLUCINATIONS

Gordon (*sensitivity psychosis*): Gordon was experiencing visual and auditory hallucinations. As is common in sensitivity psychosis, neither of these symptoms was particularly emotionally distressing, and there was no evidence of avoidance or safety behaviors. The symptoms were mostly viewed as puzzling and difficult to explain. The vague, "swirling" visual hallucinations were explained by links to the delusion of thought broadcasting, which was by far the most distressing symptom. The visual hallucinations here would respond to critical collaborative investigation of the experience itself, using a hallucinations diary (similar to the Diary of Voices in Appendix 5.4). This would allow linked triggers to be identified and hands-on investigation of the hallucination itself. Could there be a viable alternative explanation? If so, reduction of anxiety might help reduce the experience of both. This can be organized as homework. Such an intervention against the visual hallucinations would take place over three or four sessions.

Gordon's auditory hallucinations took the form of thought echoes linked to the delusion of thought broadcasting. This more troublesome symptom, which led to shame, embarrassment, and social withdrawal, often exacerbates negative symptoms. Critical collaborative investigation of the location of the voice can be followed by discussion of mechanisms. If telepathy is suggested, then this can be considered in relation to the related evidence (see the "Understanding Voices" leaflet in Appendix 4). If the thought echo occurs during a session, then an attempt might be made to tape the thoughts. A diary of voices is used to detect the fluctuations in the experience and to evaluate some of the listed coping strategies. Thought echo is extremely responsive to rational responding in which the stress that is linked to the thoughts is explored and the cognitive distortions noted. Rational responses are then placed on a cue card or audiotape in order that the thoughts can be engaged and responded to. With the techniques described above, we would expect excellent results with both the visual hallucinations and thought echo. Once learned, these techniques are usually not forgotten, and a durable effect can be achieved.

Craig (*drug-related psychosis*): Craig's voices are a much more difficult proposition. Only with a full understanding of the case formulation could the most effective techniques be generated. His voices were repeating his own thoughts and commanding him to undertake violent actions that he has previously carried out, making Craig a potential risk to himself and others. Motivational interviewing to help work toward reduced use of illegal substances would be supplemented by the use of the full range of coping strategies. It is vital to investigate a number of these systematically, as improved coping must be the first starting point. At the start of each session the current risk must be explored and recorded. A likely success experience might be achieved by using rational responding, as in Gordon's case. Work on the command hallucinations can be done in imagery using the exposure model described earlier in this chapter. This work is linked to normalizing explanations; obsessional thoughts are normal at times of stress and can be dealt with without increasing anxiety and anger that result in his lashing out. From his case formulation there should be some guidance as to which schemas are most pertinent to the maintenance of his voices. Schema-level work may assist in sustaining improvement in such a case. If there is any coexisting personality disorder, this would need to be worked upon at the schema level with appropriate exercises. This is the type of case that would need to be supervised in terms of the cognitive therapy and the work done in a setting of repeated risk assessment and multidisciplinary collaboration.

Gillian (*traumatic psychosis*): Gillian's voices are quite different again. In content and form the voices resemble flashbacks to incestuous abuse. The themes are of cleanliness, prostitution, and criticism. Linked visual images are of her brother commanding her in relation to the foregoing experiences. The reported bionic arm may have been her way of describing the unacceptable actions involved in her being used as a prostitute by her brother. Working with the voices here involved working with the distortions within the voice content and the linked images and gradually working through the disclosure of the abuse. Rational responding using a personal tape recorder and gradual exposure to the voices with experiments in response prevention eventually allowed some degree of control to be reestablished. This, in turn, enabled the voices to subside, with a greatly reduced need for antipsychotic medication in terms of dosage, thus permitting successful rehabilitation to take place. A great deal of support was needed in the setting of a clear formulation, and confident therapy over approximately 30 sessions was needed to turn this revolving-door case around. A durable and significant improvement has been achieved, and due to the reduced cost of hospitalization the cognitive therapy has been highly cost-effective.

Paul (*anxiety psychosis*): Paul's only hallucinations were thought to have occurred within the first few days of admission, when his anxiety levels were extremely high and before the delusional system had emerged. In such an acute hallucinosis cognitive therapy involves brief regular sessions of normalizing (e.g., in relation to sleep deprivation), anxiety reduction using rational responses, and relaxation with consistent explanation. Coping strategies are instituted, and information is regularly given. The voice content will probably be very useful in the case formulation, as it often relates very directly to key past events and the underlying schemas.

ELEVEN

Thought Interference, Passivity Phenomena, and Formal Thought Disorder

Thought interference and passivity phenomena are specific forms of disorder of thought content (i.e., delusions) that deserve consideration in their own right because of the techniques used to supplement those used with delusions generally. Formal thought disorder involves changes in the way thoughts are expressed.

THOUGHT INTERFERENCE

Thought interference is a common problem with people who are oversensitive to the world around them. It is often associated with delusions of reference. The feeling that people are talking about you, usually critically, and even know what you are thinking is very intrusive and unpleasant. Thought broadcasting, in particular, represents a most intimate invasion of your person. In this instance, the person is convinced that other people know of his or her thoughts and that he or she can do nothing to stop it. All the person can do is to try not to think or at least keep their thoughts "clean and wholesome"—and even the effort to do so is thought to make this goal impossible.

As with all delusional beliefs, getting back to the start—the first time this occurred—is the first step in understanding it. However, because the nature of the thoughts may be embarrassing, the person may well frustrate the therapist's attempts to do this—at least until a good relationship has been established. It is often more productive to deal with these specific symptoms by analyzing recent occurrences and setting up ways of examining them in the future.

"Has it happened recently?"

"Where were you?"

"Can you describe to me exactly what happened?"

It is then important to elicit:

"Who did you think knew what you were thinking?"

"Why did they think that?"

"What was it you were thinking at the time?"

If the client hesitates, it may be worth adding:

"I don't need to know exactly what you thought, but was it unpleasant or just some mundane thoughts?"

It may be worth exploring possible consequences as you build up the picture of a number of instances of this happening:

"Were there any consequences to this seeming to happen?"

"Why did you yourself think it was happening?"

"Was anything happening in your life at the time?"

You may be able to ask the person directly if he or she felt under stress or not, but if the person's delusional conviction is very high this may simply be taken as your not believing them. So, it is probably better to avoid being too specific unless the person has previously related it to stress. However, it usually does not harm to ask "Is there any pattern to this happening?" This can be explored—sometimes there is an obvious pattern, sometimes not. This is an obvious point at which to introduce a diary, if you think it may be completed (see examples in Appendix 5). Certainly passing out a copy of the leaflet titled "Understanding What Others Think" (from Appendix 4) with a diary, "as an example of something which you might find useful," gives your clients the option of using it if they wish without their "failing" if they don't.

Once you have identified one or more specific instances and reviewed the person's understanding of it, it may be possible to explore the meanings of what occurred. There will often be a specific behavior exhibited by the person who they think knows the clients thoughts—for example, they laugh or look at the person or speak to someone with them—or a combination of these—or they may say something, which may be on radio or television, that relates in some way to what the person has thought. To confuse matters further, the client may be experiencing auditory hallucinations, echoing, or commenting on what they are thinking, which they then attribute to others. Disentangling this can be tricky, but concentrating on whom the client believes at that moment is "hearing" him or her is usually the best place to begin.

If the client begins with the belief that his or her thoughts are being broadcast, the behavior he or she observes is often sufficient to confirm this to him or her. The therapeutic goal is to enable the client to look at alternatives to this possibility; for example, you might ask:

"Do you think there are any other ways of understanding what happened?"

"Could they have been laughing at somebody else? Or at a joke one of them had made?" (Usually this is not convincing!)

Switching to discussing how it happens can begin to open up other possibilities:

"How do you think they know your thoughts?"

Explanations may be vague but sometimes involve a general belief, which may or may not be construed as a conspiracy, that reading minds is a perfectly normal thing that everyone but the client is capable of doing. Alternatively, it may be just selected people who can do this—people in the Secret Service, witches, or the like. One client described his belief in the phenomenon of brain waves that are transmitted like sound or light waves from electrical currents in the brain and that certain highly sensitive people can detect and understand. It is at this point, quite often, that a discussion of telepathy becomes relevant:

"Do you mean something like telepathy?"

Many people find this a way of explaining what they experience that allows for a common language to emerge and then to be debated. Many simply let out a sigh of relief that, at last, somebody can understand what they are talking about. This, of course, does not mean that you are validating their conclusion, but at least you are opening up this line of communication. If the client does find the analogy to telepathy useful, it is possible to discuss what people mean by telepathy and the experiments that have been done to investigate it, commencing by exploring his or her understanding of the concept:

"So, do you know anything about telepathy?"

Most people can give a brief description. They may give examples of close family members who believe that they have been able to communicate with each other without words—that is, know what someone is thinking before they do or say it, or instantly sense a traumatic event occurring to a close family member miles away. It is often helpful to elaborate this further:

"There have been experiments to see if people can communicate telepathically. Beginning as early as the 1960s, scientists would get people to sit in one room and look at playing cards or the like to see whether their counterparts in another room could correctly name which cards they had looked at. On balance, some people appeared to consistently perform better than average on such tests of "extrasensory perception," or ESP. There are various possible explanations for this.[1] But there certainly didn't seem to be any evidence that people could read someone else's train of thoughts—even when renowned psychics were tested."

It is possible to object to this line of reasoning, arguing that perhaps conditions have to be "right" for telepathy to occur and experimental conditions may interfere with it. But what seems most important is the frank discussion of these phenomena so that—just as

[1]For example, the tendency for positive studies to be more likely to be published than negative ones. This may be too complicated an explanation for most persons to be useful to them, but it could be useful for some.

you demonstrate that a critical approach has been taken to these phenomena—so can the person him- or herself examine them.

Often a discussion of nonverbal communication is relevant. Sometimes the client seems to lack an understanding of nonverbal communication altogether, or to misconceive its nature. So, when the person thinks there is some form of communication going on that excludes him or her, the client interprets it as thought transmission. He or she may be aware of "knowing" smiles and other gestures possibly from family members or staff or friends but may be unable to recognize them for what they really are, or fully understand them. Simple explanations may involve the discussion of, for example, how one's tone of voice, gestures, body movements, facial expressions, and eye contact can reflect emotions and meaning.

Personal examples work best—if possible, from your own interaction with the person or your observed behavior of others. As usual, the most effective way of understanding this is through drawing out knowledge from the person rather than through "teaching" him or her:

> "Do you think it might have had something to do with the way they laughed that made you think they'd read your thoughts?"

> "Was it a bit sarcastic, or were they looking directly at you—making eye contact—when they did it?"

> "Eye contact is quite often used to ensure that someone has understood what you are saying or doing or that you have heard them."

More often than not, the client is looking away or does so rapidly, so he or she cannot readily confirm eye contact. It may then be that asking them to "keep watch" can help. Far from making them more paranoid, it usually makes them more critical of what they see and more open to alternative explanations.

Changes in these symptoms can occur quite quickly, but direct confrontation of them may not be helpful—repeated measuring of degree of conviction, for example, may have the effect of entrenching it. Thought broadcasting is often directly related to other symptoms and recedes as mood lifts and confidence builds.

Thought withdrawal is more uncommon and may relate to thought block. When someone is anxious and self-conscious, sometimes the person's train of thought may be interrupted and he or she comes to a standstill. In fact, it is only the train of thought that is blocked—other thoughts flood in: "help, what was I thinking about? . . . where has it gone? . . . oh, come on . . . try and remember . . . I'm so stupid . . . " This may be interpreted as thoughts being taken or withdrawn, especially when the person is suspicious of interference occurring to him or her. Relating the beliefs to thought block and a little self-disclosure of times when you've experienced it or known someone else who experienced it may be relevant—for example, during public speaking. Discussing the mechanisms is useful:

> "Who could or would have wanted to withdraw your thoughts?"

> "How could they do it?"

This may just elicit uncertainty—or specific delusional beliefs such as, for example:

"It is the CIA—they've been experimenting on people like me to test it out in the Middle East."

Such beliefs can then be examined and understood in the way that we have described therapeutic work with delusions (see Chapter 9).

Thought insertion also seems quite uncommon and is essentially a "made" thought—one believed to be of someone else's construction. There may be a variety of explanations for their occurrence, but many relate to automatic thoughts occurring that are sexual or violent or otherwise embarrassing. The belief may be that these thoughts couldn't originate from the person's own mind—"I couldn't think something so bad"— and so they must have been put there by someone else. A possible alternative to this is that these thoughts are perceived as "voices" (see Chapter 10). As with work with such voices, discussion of the existence and nature of automatic thoughts may assist the person in accepting ownership of the thoughts while retaining the differentiation between having thoughts and acting upon them.

Thought echo, again, is relatively uncommon. In our experience, it again relates to the ownership of thoughts—people come to realize that there is a flow of thoughts that proceeds whether they like it or not. To a large extent, these thoughts happen spontaneously and can be difficult to control. They may come to seem to be something that is an echo of what the person thinks and are often more distracting than distressing. Understanding and learning to live with them become the goal. Isolation and limited activity reinforce the phenomenon, so work on associated negative symptoms can help in the longer term.

PASSIVITY PHENOMENA

Feeling that others or some external agency or force is making you do, think, or feel things—not just psychologically coercing you—must be profoundly disturbing and disempowering. Such things can be what the person particularly does not want to do but sometimes are things that they would like to be able to do but that they recognize to be wrong. The "made" feelings can be unpleasant or simply annoying or irritating. Such "made" thoughts as those discussed above can be similar, if not identical, to thought insertion. Understanding such passivity phenomena may be assisted by the case formulation.

> Without any apparent provocation, Ken rushed around and broke down his neighbor's door. He returned to his own house, denied any responsibility for this action, and described himself as feeling powerless to stop it. His childhood had been disrupted by the death of his mother, and he had lived with a number of different aunts and uncles since then. He was very shy and had never formed any close relationships. It emerged that, among a number of other factors, for many years he had felt envious of his neighbor's good relationship with others, and the action may have been a reaction to this.

It may be that the phenomena are components of a broader psychotic picture; for example, "made" feelings may link with visual or auditory hallucinations and feelings of fear when related at original onset to hallucinogenic drug experiences. They may be part of overwhelming emotional experiences and "disowned" following them—for example, a belief that the neighbors are interfering in your life may lead to your smashing their window. Passivity may often be in response to voices—voices that are believed to be all-powerful—and this, in turn, can lead to acting on what they say—because the person believes he or she has no choice in the matter.

The therapist and client should carefully assess the times when passivity is operating, identify the first time it occurred, and then a discussion of possible mechanisms can follow.

"What do you think made you do [or feel, or think] that?"

"Was it some sort of physical force—for example, hypnotism or magnetism?"

"Or did it have to do with who you think is the source of the voice (e.g., the devil or God)?"

If some specific physical force is involved, discussion of such forces may be relevant. Hypnotism is quite common as an explanation. Inquiry into how the client thought he or she was induced into a hypnotic trance can be fruitful. It certainly seems to be the case that induction cannot occur without consent and indeed active participation.

"When did you think you were induced into a hypnotic state?"

"If you can't remember, why do you think that is?"

"We could look into this further, but my understanding is that you couldn't be hypnotized without participating in that initial process."

This may be something that the person wants to find further information about. Similarly, exploration of beliefs about other forces can examine whether they could exert the sort of influence that the person thinks they do.

When voices are the source of commands, issues of omnipotence need to be addressed (see Chapter 10). The therapist should suggest to the client that just because voices may sound loud and powerful does not mean that what they say is true or has to be obeyed—any more than anyone else shouting that they must do something. The distinction between the words and actions is essential to make—"just because they tell you to hurt yourself or someone else doesn't mean you have to do it!"

"If I shouted at you 'Give me all your money,' would you have to do that?"

"So, why should you do what the voices say?"

The client may respond that the voices or whoever is the source of the order has power—for example, God will be angry if he or she does not respond and will punish him or her. Discussion of such spiritual beliefs is covered elsewhere (see Chapter 9). The fear of punishment can be a significant and distressing—and self-fulfilling—phenomenon. Sometimes demonstrating contradictions can help—"Do you always do what is said or not always?" (Usually they haven't; sometimes they have been punished—but often not.) Or you may be able to help the client cope with any increase in voices or other distress in some way. Responses to commands do tend to be more common where the risk or threatened damage is less and much less where the risk is more serious.

As with most delusional ideas, these discussions can open up a dialogue and a general approach based on the formulation allows such beliefs to gradually recede in importance and reduce the associated distress.

THOUGHT DISORDER

Based on the cognitive model of thought disorder (described in Chapter 1), the key goal of therapy for thought disorder is to assist the person in communicating so that he or she can be understood. Without achieving this, both assessment and case formulation become very difficult. This may mean that work on thought disorder becomes the primary concern to enable therapy for other symptoms to proceed.

Emotional disturbance may be a significant feature of thought disorder. Often, as emotionally salient areas are reached in discussions, so thought disorder worsens. It may seem to act as a screen around these areas and then a diversion from them. This can assist assessment when recognized, but does mean that a different approach route may be needed. Thought disorder may be related to substance misuse, particularly with "hallucinogenics"—amphetamines, cocaine, ecstasy, LSD, and sometimes cannabis. Use of these substances is often correlated with an increased rate of speech and distractibility. Thought disorder can also sometimes seem to be a process by which interaction occurs with others in a nonthreatening way—almost becoming a conversational style. It can seem to be teasing: "Let's see if you can make out what I'm saying—are you really prepared to try, or are you going to simply dismiss me, as others do?" Sometimes there can seem to be an air of grandiosity about thought disorder: "I am unique and speak in this unique fashion—in fact, it is a hyper-intelligent language. Just see if you can understand me." Trying to do so—looking for the use of metaphor or other clues to meaning—can therefore not only help communication but sometimes be profoundly rapport-developing (even quite good fun—but may be rather like completing difficult crossword puzzles!).

Initial Goals

So, it is always important to demonstrate a willingness to try to understand your client. The client will usually also realize that communication between the two of you is a necessary goal. It may not at this point be appropriate to be explicit about the possible reasons for the thought disorder. Often it is premature to do so before completing a full formulation, although working on communication may be necessary before such a formulation is developed. At a later stage, a discussion of the reasons for thought disorder may be appropriate, although this may seem unnecessary—discussing the means for communicating rather than the underlying issues themselves. Discussing how you will try to understand may be reasonable, but just doing it is essential!

Disentangling Thought Disorder

Developing order out of disorder involves gently structuring conversation. So, initially—as with all therapeutic encounters—allowing a flow of conversation to occur is necessary in enabling the person to express his or her point of view and their particular favored issues. It may not be clear to you what that point of view is nor what issues are favored, but it is worth trying to understand and suggest possibilities. In other words, make an educated guess on what you know of the person so far—linked to any key words that he or she has said they say. Key words generally would include emotionally charged terms—"she died," "major accident," "so painful," "shut up." Any "guess" needs to be short and to the point—"Do you mean your mother?" or "Are you referring to an accident that's happened to you?"

Responses can vary from annoyance or anger, to "Listen!," to simply ignoring what you've said, or to an acknowledgement, "Yes, my mother." It may take time to begin to draw out important themes with repetition—that is, asking for clarification:

> "I didn't really understand what you meant by 'hellification,' although it sounds unpleasant."

The pace of work depends on the person's responses. If what you say is irritating him or her—say, to the extent of the client's threatening to leave—you may simply have to sit and allow what he or she says to wash over you until the person comes to a stop or asks you something or slows down sufficiently to allow you to begin again. However, usually people welcome your help in clarifying their difficulties in communicating. They will allow you to focus on a particular topic and to question them gently about it. This may take the form of closed questions (with yes or no answers) initially, opening up as the topic develops. It may even be possible to keep them on topic through interruptions:

> "Do you think we can just finish talking about original topic before moving on to talk about that?"

This should be done lightheartedly, if possible, which softens the intervention:

> "Whoa . . . Hold on a minute . . . Let's just see if I can understand first what [e.g., your concern about the FBI] is all about . . . I'm a bit slow today!"

Frequently you will reach a point at which further clarification is not proving successful and may then move on, remembering to return to the topic later that session or in a future one. Quite often what appears to be an important route turns out to be a blind alley, but the process of focusing conversation often helps in exploring more relevant areas. It does involve the therapists having faith that there is meaning in the depths of the conversation—and that can be hard to find in the more profoundly thought-disordered person. However, given time, some order always seems to emerge—thought disorder may be biologically influenced, but some of it, at least, can still make sense.

Involving others close to the person—caregivers, staff, and friends—can reinforce this ordering of communication. So often, those who know the person best understand what is being referred to and may well act as interpreters for you. Moreover, as they observe you extracting some sense from the ostensible verbal chaos, they will often strive to find it themselves (see Figure 11.1).

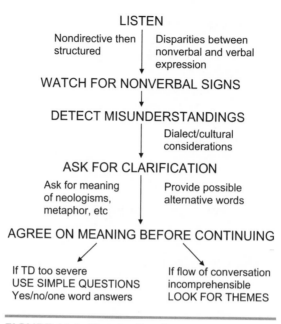

FIGURE 11.1. Thought disorder: Techniques for clarifying verbal communication.

THOUGHT INTERFERENCE, PASSIVITY PHENOMENA, AND THOUGHT DISORDER

Gordon (*sensitivity psychosis*): Thought interference has been a key issue for Gordon. He has a persisting belief that others can read his thoughts but he can't read theirs. Sometimes he can identify a particular time and person who is doing this, but usually he views it as a more general issue. Some of this seemed to be explained by a misunderstanding of the way nonverbal communication occurs, and so this was discussed at some length and he agreed to consult some books detailing the problem. Although not entirely convinced, the reading has made this a less intrusive belief, and Gordon is less fearful about going out. In particular, he has felt able to go to crowded places (e.g., sports events), which previously he found overwhelming. He also had issues with passivity—in particular, a feeling of pressure in his stomach that he could not understand but that seemed to be external in origin. Again, discussion of the effects of anxiety and stress has been used to provide an explanatory framework for him. This has enabled him to accept a possible internal cause for it—so he now wants a body scan done!

Craig (*drug-related psychosis*): Thought disorder has intruded into Craig's conversations, particularly when he was acutely ill, but generally it has been possible to communicate by checking the meanings of phrases used that were difficult to understand. As this has improved, it has become clearer that Craig has passivity phenomena associated with voices and "flashbacks." He feels as though he is being physically pushed around, and again these feelings of tension seem related to episodes when he is particularly anxious and psychotic symptoms develop. Again, exploring the relationship between these symptoms and stress is gradually being accepted.

Gillian (*traumatic psychosis*): At times, Gillian wondered whether her thoughts could be read by others, but she was relatively easily dissuaded from this opinion. However, her belief that she could be made to do things, especially harm herself, by the voices could be very strong. This was tackled with reattribution, discussing content, and particularly looking at the relationship between thoughts and actions. Gillian firmly believed that she had to do what the voices said or there would be devastating consequences—although she was also able to see that, in contradiction to this, sometimes she had not done what they had said—especially the more extreme actions—and there had not been the predicted consequences (although the voices had continued to distress her). Also, when she had done what they said, this had not reduced their severity, although a transient increase in distress would occur when she resisted. Work on the perceived power of the voices was therefore of great importance and took time.

Paul (*anxiety psychosis*): Thought interference, disorder, or passivity did not feature in Paul's presentation.

TWELVE

Negative Symptoms

Negative symptoms induce negativity in therapists, caregivers, and people with schizophrenia. These symptoms (see Table 12.1) just seem to defy understanding and certainly solution. Whatever you try, things appear impervious to change. If anything they just go on getting worse and worse, and you get more and more demoralized, so they get worse still. "Burnout" may not be far off—and reaching a point at which you say "I can do no more" may even be a relief. But it does not need to be like that.

There is now evidence that psychological treatment can make a difference to negative symptoms. Our study (Sensky et al., 2000) showed sustained and substantial improvement in negative symptoms—and while befriending was taking place this also helped although its effect was reduced afterward. Neil Rector's group similarly produced a significant positive effect in their study (Rector et al., 2003) as did Pinto and colleagues (Pinto et al., 1999). Nick Tarrier and colleagues (2001) also showed changes that were close to significance.

This cognitive model (Kingdon & Turkington, 1994) of the emergence of primary negative symptoms (alogia, affective blunting, and autism) echoes the work of Bleuler (1911). Bleuler viewed these as being the primary symptoms of schizophrenia (along with ambivalence and disturbance of association) and suggested that they represented

TABLE 12.1. Brief Descriptions of Negative Symptoms

Affective flattening	Decreased and less responsive facial and vocal expressiveness and reduced eye contact.
Alogia	Slowness to respond; amount and content of speech restricted or interrupted.
Avolition	Limited in general activity, including personal care, schooling, or work.
Anhedonia	Feeling of emptiness and reduced interest in activities and relationships.
Social withdrawal	Reduced participation in relationships (e.g., with friends and family) and active withdrawal.
Attention deficit	Difficulty in concentrating and remembering.

TABLE 12.2. Cognitive Therapy Explanations for Negative Symptoms

Affective flattening	Sometimes equivalent to shock, it may develop from demoralization, perhaps related to past traumatic events, perhaps defensive in character.
Alogia	Is it lack of thoughts or difficulty in communicating? Could it be a reaction to criticism?
Avolition	Possibly "driven to a standstill" by the perception of being under pressure and subject to failing expectations.
Anhedonia	Hopeless, numbed, and demoralized.
Social withdrawal	A mechanism to reduce stress by lowering overstimulation.
Attention deficit	Overstimulated, causing poor concentration and attention.

a defensive position in relation to unbearable levels of stress. Such symptoms may indeed be more common in people with high levels of vulnerability and a low capacity to cope with stress, who often develop social phobia, agoraphobia, and tendencies toward institutionalization. Table 12.2 lists the cognitive therapy explanations for various negative symptoms.

It has long been known that this group of clients may gradually "warm up" with gentle supportive psychotherapy. Cognitive therapy can be useful by using a gentle, slow conversational style with activity scheduling, using paradoxically low targets— "taking the pressure off." Clients may slowly begin to recognize these issues and work with coping with stress. They may then begin to allow more work with any coexisting phobic symptoms that are often exacerbated by delusions of reference or thought broadcasting. Negative symptoms can be improved with parallel work on coexisting positive symptoms, initially focusing on those that are less emotionally charged. As the person begins to develop confidence, he or she then begins to make decisions that lead to less withdrawal and more engagement in social and employment settings. This model provides a firm foundation on which to build therapeutic strategies.

CONVALESCENCE

After an acute initial episode or a relapse, it may take time for recovery—psychological healing—to occur. The experience itself will have been seriously traumatizing for most people with schizophrenia. The symptoms themselves, even when resolved, will have been confusing and distressing. They may lack meaning, or have very disturbing meanings, and recovery involves trying to understand—and that takes time. The contact with mental health services, which involves seeing a psychiatrist and possibly even admission to the hospital, will have been unexpected and at times is so traumatic as to be described as producing symptoms of posttraumatic stress disorder. The new perception of the self as a "mentally ill person" (as the client may have previously regarded anybody with mental health problems) may take awhile to assimilate.

Strauss (1989) has described the "woodshedding" analogy of the jazz musician who goes down to the shed at the bottom of the garden to compose a new piece for performance. To the outside world, nothing much may seem to be happening—apart from a cacophony of sound—until finally the musician emerges, rehearsed and ready to per-form. Interrupting him, pestering him to engage in other activities, and generally inter-fering with his practice just increases the time needed and may even prevent him from being ready to perform. Similarly, with people with schizophrenia who are trying to re-cover, it may be better *not* to strive too hard to help, or to persuade them to go to day centers, or to return to work, or to go out to see friends. Simply being available when needed may be the best way to help. Letting them recover in their own good time at their own pace is probably essential.

Another analogy that caregivers and people with schizophrenia have found help-ful is that of a broken leg. Such an injury needs rest, protection, and time to heal—usu-ally less time than after an acute psychotic episode. But taking it out of a plaster cast too early or not immobilizing it in plaster in the first place just builds up problems for the future. Similarly, immobilization—or at least peaceful relaxation—is needed to heal a mind that has been traumatized. Even years after an episode in which negative symp-toms have predominated, the concept of a period of convalescence can still be valuable and destigmatizing.

THE PROTECTIVE NATURE OF NEGATIVE SYMPTOMS

Negative symptoms have gotten a bad name—at times, inappropriately. Actually, in practice, they can be highly protective. Social withdrawal, for example, may reduce stress and positive symptoms. When the person is in his or her room alone, voices may be less insistent—or at least they can talk to the person without disturbing others. So-cial contact at this time may be difficult—particularly if it provokes delusions of refer-ence and thought broadcasting. No people, no such delusions.

Many people with schizophrenia shift their waking hours so that they get up late and go to bed during the early-morning hours. The sedative effects of medication may make it difficult to rise early, but it is equally true that the early-morning hours can be quite stressful. Other members of the household may be leaving for work, reinforcing the fact that the client isn't. They may also be highly irritable, and it may simply be too stimulating an environment—everyone bustling about the kitchen, radios and TVs blaring, arguments about being late for work or school, and so forth. Avoiding all of this may make great sense, and the very early hours of the morning—between mid-night and 3 A.M.—can be peaceful and relaxing.

Before dealing with such protective "negative" symptoms, therapeutic work with relevant positive symptoms may be needed to reduce the chance of their flaring up or to provide ways of managing the stress that may precede them—or to have coping strategies ready for their onset. The ability to tolerate stress better is almost always a necessary intermediate-term goal.

NEGATIVE SYMPTOM PRESENTATIONS

As mentioned earlier, premorbid development is important in assessing management. If poor, as demonstrated by underachievement in school (that is, frequently at the bot-tom or near the bottom of the class) and social isolation, the approach may need to be broader and involve greater emphasis on developing general social and other skills than where premorbid development has been good or adequate. If school attainments have been average or good, possibly even to the college level, work with expectations is likely to be particularly important. With in the latter group, typically social development is quite variable, and therefore assessment and attention should be directed toward identified areas of deficit.

Within the former group, that is, those evidencing poor premorbid development, skills development may well be very important though sometimes quite difficult because of poor morale and a low level of ability. Emotional skills, for example, anxiety management, assertiveness, and emotion recognition training, will be needed, along with basic literacy work and other social skills development. These clients may well have difficulties coping with the demands of daily living, social interaction, and certainly employment.

With the group with better premorbid development, reducing immediate pressures and expectations may be the first step toward making progress. "Convalescence," as noted earlier, may be needed even years after the most recent acute episode—so that the person can relax and "get his (or her) head together."

PLANNING MANAGEMENT

Setting Treatment Goals

Agreeing on the goals of treatment would seem to be particularly important in view of the previous discussions about identifying and achieving expectations. However, even the discussion of "What are we aiming for?" can sometimes induce panic and certainly the perception of pressure in the person. Therefore, it is very important to proceed initially only with short-term goals and defer specific discussion of long-term goals, or at least keep them very general—for example, "for things to improve." So, the approach might be:

> "It's important that you rest and relax. Let's take the pressure off, and that's all we'll aim for at the moment."

> "When you're relaxed and feeling better, then we can start thinking about the future."

For most people with schizophrenia, that is all the discussion of goals that is needed at this stage. Some will want to discuss goals in more detail, and certainly caregivers frequently will. Probably the best approach is to suggest, for example, that:

> "We'll just put things on hold for the moment. It doesn't mean that you can't try to go to college in the future [or "go back to your course or job"], but let's just take it one step at a time."

In the person's mind and that of his caregivers, there are goals—usually explicit—that are waiting to be achieved (see Figure 12.1).

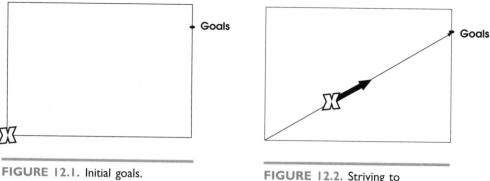

FIGURE 12.1. Initial goals.

FIGURE 12.2. Striving to achieve goals.

Achievement of the goals may be attempted directly (see Figure 12.2).

Or, the client may try to reach his or her goals even more quickly than expected or planned (see Figure 12.3)!

However, actual performance often does not live up to expectations. Instead of achieving the goals, the person bumps along the bottom, repeatedly failing and actually achieving less and less (see Figure 12.4).

A gentler route that is more likely to be successful would be that shown in Figure 12.5. The initial aim would be to achieve very little apart from just feeling better, in and of itself. Once this is achieved and the person feels able to recommence activities such as studying, working, or social interaction, a very gentle introduction is needed, after which he or she can than control the pace of activity.

Such an approach may initially involve reducing the level of activity if the person feels particularly poorly motivated and demoralized, but with time the person can recommence under his or her own initiative and control (see Figure 12.6).

It may even be that resetting goals at a lower level will be needed (see Figure 12.7), but this is not usually the first step. It is only if it becomes clear after a few months or years that the goals need to be revised and are overambitious in the long-term that this

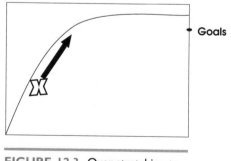

FIGURE 12.3. Over-stretching to achieve goals.

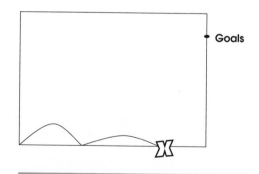

FIGURE 12.4. Failure and demoralization.

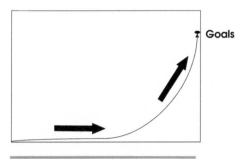

FIGURE 12.5. Achieving expectations.

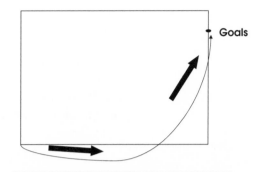

FIGURE 12.6. Achieving expectations by initially reducing pressure.

possibility should be discussed. The aim is to develop and eventually achieve agreed-upon goals. If symptoms have been present less than a year, the timetable normally involves months. If symptoms have been present, say, for a number of years, recovery may also take a number of years. We often start by suggesting "taking a year off" and then "seeing how you are getting on then." This does not mean that the therapist will necessarily spend a great deal of time with the client over that year or two—infrequent sessions (say, every three to four weeks) may be quite appropriate. The true gains in resource management, come through reducing hospitalization time.

Importance and Nature of Effective Treatment Goals

As has become apparent, setting goals is tricky but essential. The goals certainly need to be mutually agreed-upon but without causing the client to feel unduly pressured in the here and now. Some goals may seem conventional and obvious and need little exploration—such matters as finding a satisfying job, a home of your own, some good trusty friends, and a long-term partner. But, of course, not every person will subscribe

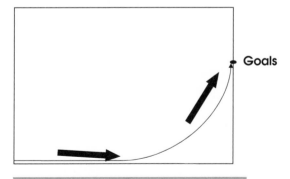

FIGURE 12.7. Achieving expectations with revision of long-term goals.

to these goals, and many may have alternatives. For some, spirituality and ethical matters (for example, environmental conservation) may be prominent ends in themselves, and they may form specific goals in these areas. Living alone may be perfectly acceptable as a goal. A job that is not particularly satisfying but allows plenty of time to do other things or pays very well may be a person's objective. However, for people with schizophrenia presenting with negative symptoms, these are usually relatively distant goals. They can be explored to the degree that does not distress the person, but it may be more appropriate to leave them as vague directions to be firmed up as time permits. Frequently the person will give hints of their own personal goals spontaneously—for example:

"I wish I had some friends."

"If only I could get back into that training course!"

Short-term goals are important to set but need to be readily and consistently achievable. If the initial goals are not achieved, they need to be reset to reduce the effort required so that they can be. So that they will be limited and pressure-reducing. It may be enough to advise:

"Just take it easy, relax, and recuperate."

"How about getting up for a cup of tea mid-morning and then going back to bed?"

"Could you make it to the shops yourself to get your cigarettes rather than have your mother get them?"

These are common initial short-term goals to set. Only once the person him- or herself is ready do you start to discuss, let alone set, goals that are more demanding. These may then be to do something very simple—ideally suggested by the person him- or herself. It is often a good tactic to advise that, whatever is suggested, he or she does less. This is because often the person strives for too much too quickly, and reducing the pressure, ensuring success, as far as possible, is a more effective way of achieving joint goals. As the person begins to reach for goals, he or she may begin to fear the experience of discomfort or distress. This may take the form of an increase in hallucinations or the experience of delusions of reference, and/or increased anxiety that may feel intense or to which he or she may have developed a low tolerance.

Intermediate-term goals can gradually be developed as short-term goals are consistently achieved. For example, returning to work may be out of the question, but going to a social event—for example, a brother's wedding or a drop-in group—may be possible. The trip to the drop-in group may require more motivation than the family event, and bridging the client's confidence gap will usually be necessary—for example, with mental health worker accompanying and staying for a first visit, at least. It will also depend on how well the group is functioning, how welcoming it is, and whether others with common interests also attend. If the group doesn't suit your client's purposes, don't push the issue unduly. If you seem to disapprove of or show disappointment with the client's reaction, the client may feel that he or she has failed you, others, and themselves, and slip back rather than stay in neutral. It will be that much longer before he or she is willing to consider a step forward again. There may need to be regular readjustment of goals as necessary.

When the time comes, long-term "5-year plans" may be drawn up and referred to, as needed, to help combat demoralization. Maintaining hope is an essential component of therapy that can be instilled by having limited but specific goals and sometimes by discussing more general but less specific broad objectives. For example:

> "Just because we're agreeing that you need to rest and relax now doesn't mean that you can't become a rocket scientist in the future. . . . It's just best at the moment to concentrate on living day-to-day and feeling better about yourself. We may need to consider what you do want to do in the future, but we don't have to do it today."

Even though—or perhaps especially because—long-term objectives and intermediate-term goals evolve over time and may not be detailed immediately, and short-term goals can be described in relatively imprecise terms, this does not mean that the therapist can have imprecise goals and objectives. Individualized goals need to be set and standardized methods used for assessing the goals. This can be through the use of standardized instruments—for example, measuring a decline in anxiety or distress from hallucinations, which is probably safest when therapists are training and new to the role (see Chapter 5). Evaluating symptoms in a nonstandardized but clinically sensitive way also be effective. That is, people with schizophrenia may be asked about their mood, stress, and voices: How bad are their episodes? How frequent are they? How interfering? The answer will be dependent on the presenting symptoms. When goals become more concrete, the number of times the person goes out, the distance from home, and/or the amount of social contact they experience can all be used as appropriate measures of progress.

The initial treatment plan derived from the case formulation will include references to negative symptoms but also include other areas that may impact upon them. Psychoeducation, especially into the nature of negative symptoms and the explanations for them, is a core part of therapy (see Figure 12.8). There is a need to reduce pressure and expectations to manageable levels and to explain the theory behind it. Leaflets (such as those in Appendix 4) may help as a guide for the client, caregiver, and therapist.

"Pressure points"—specific sources of stress—need to be identified by using guided discovery. This will often come out during discussion of the presenting problems and their development but may need confirmation or may need to be directly elicited:

> "So, going down to the corner shop is a real problem, is that right? . . . What about supermarkets or shops farther away from home?"

The key principle is that:

> *You can't push people out of negative symptoms.*

But you may be able to help them find and open doors.

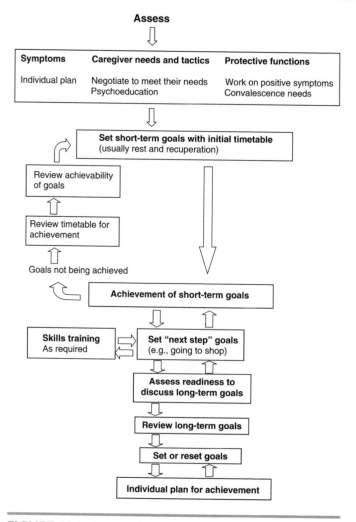

FIGURE 12.8. Flow diagram for negative symptoms.

WORKING WITH FAMILIES, CAREGIVERS, AND STAFF

Negative symptoms cause caregivers more concern than any other symptoms. They are difficult to understand and have practical implications for the caregivers. It is easy to believe that such symptoms are due to laziness or certainly willfulness in some way and can thus be characterized by the caregiver as "critical expressed emotion." It also means that others have to contribute more to domestic and to tasks to compensate, causing resentment in caregivers, family members, and, if at work, colleagues. However, much of the concern derives from these beliefs rather than the actual consequences. Being able to discuss the existence and nature of negative symptoms as part of schizophrenia is a useful first step in accepting, understanding, and managing them. Frequently caregivers try to help by striving to motivate the person—pushing and applying psychological pressure—on the basis that this will push-start activity. However, this effort becomes counterproductive, and discussion initiated by the therapist—that, while his or her intentions are good, the tactics might need review—can reduce distress on all sides.

Some caregivers do find "letting go" and stepping back very difficult, but many are relieved at being told that they can do so. Those who find it difficult can often be persuaded of the logic for so doing. But the habit may die hard, and reducing contact with the person or having another caregiver as intermediary may be the only way, at least in the first instance, to handle that situation. With progress, however, the message often gets across and is accepted.

Some negative symptoms—for example, time shift—can cause other concerns. For example, playing music at 2 A.M. may not be appreciated by others living in the person's home, and negotiation over this (e.g., the use of headphones or turning the volume down) may be necessary. Caregivers may also be concerned about safety issues (e.g., smoking cigarettes causing fires), and again working out a reasonable safe compromise may be part of the treatment plan. The very fact that the person is not getting up for a working day may cause concern, but at least initially this concern can be allayed by use of a "convalescence" model:

> "In time, getting up for work or college will be necessary, but for the moment recuperation, rest, and recovery are more important."

MEDICATION REGIMES

Medication management can either enhance or interfere with progress with negative symptoms. The evidence of the effectiveness of older "typical" antipsychotics with such symptoms is very limited. The newer drugs, especially clozapine, may be able to assist, however. But it certainly seems the case that medication can interfere through the effect of sedation in slowing the person down and reducing drive, as well as extrapyramidal symptoms that cause stiffness and slowness in movement, including facial expressions. There may be a trade-off between the effectiveness of medication in reducing positive symptoms and increasing negative symptoms. Certainly reducing medication to optimal levels is necessary. This may mean running the risk of a person's symptoms increasing but, so long as the adjustment is made carefully and collaboratively (see Chapter 14 on relapse prevention), it can produce substantial gains.

NEGATIVE SYMPTOMS

Gordon (*sensitivity psychosis*): Motivation was the primary issue, and each session after initial assessment included work on this area. Early work involved his parents in the discussion of strategy and tactics. The strategy was clear—to help Gordon find and develop a career and relationships. The tactics to be used were more debatable, but both his parents and Gordon accepted that focusing on short-term achievements, such as passing college exams, was simply not possible. A period of "time-out" was needed, and a year was determined to be appropriate. As that time has passed, Gordon's moods and concentration have improved, and he got initially part-time and then almost full-time employment after completing a job preparation course. The interaction between positive symptoms and negative symptoms has been a particular area to keep under review, as the former could easily upset this progressive movement toward work and the attendant pressures it involves.

Craig (*drug-related psychosis*): Negative symptoms certainly feature as a part of Craig's problems, but the intensity of the positive symptoms also entails immediate work. Nonetheless, discussion has centered on future goals and friendships but with avoidance of inappropriate expectations or pressure.

Gillian (*traumatic psychosis*): Positive symptoms dominated the early picture for Gillian, and these were appropriately the focus of intervention. As these became more manageable, negative symptoms became more apparent. However, the latter were predominantly related to dependency and limited coping strategies that long predated her illness. Nevertheless, these became a very important focus for rehabilitation, as they were major limitations on her ability to sustain (for the first time) independent living—albeit even though the long-term aim was for rehabilitation to be within a supported environment.

Paul (*anxiety psychosis*): On presentation, negative symptoms were not a major feature, but with Paul's hospitalization and the impact of depressive and paranoid symptoms, their development became a real possibility. Prompt management therefore was necessary to avoid their emergence. Work included sessions with Paul's caregivers and good case management—reducing the secondary effects of illness.

THIRTEEN

Comorbid Conditions

PSYCHIATRIC COMORBIDITY

Psychoses commonly—perhaps usually—present as just one of a number of psychiatric diagnoses. Common accompanying diagnoses include the following:

- Substance misuse
- Personality disorders
- Anxiety, panic, and phobic disorders (including social phobia)
- Obsessive–compulsive disorder (OCD)
- Depression

Sometimes debates can occur about which diagnosis is more appropriate, schizophrenia or, for example, depression or personality disorder—or indeed any of these. Differentiation can be difficult; social phobia can merge with paranoia, OCD with hallucinations, or borderline personality disorder with schizoaffective psychosis. Figure 5.1 (p. 63) illustrates this. Management of these comorbidities where psychosis complicates the diagnosis involves initial management of the psychosis—primarily reattribution of voices and beliefs—and with achievement of this, management of the comorbid disorder. Biological treatments can sometimes benefit from using a hierarchical structure of diagnosis in which treatment of organic conditions is primary, followed by treatment of schizophrenia, then depression, and finally anxiety. Biological treatment of the higher-order diagnoses also improves those lower down. For example, antipsychotic medication often improves depressive and anxiety symptoms in psychotic disorders. However, with psychological treatment, each problem warrants addressing in its own right. So, treating positive and negative symptoms of schizophrenia may help with anxiety and depression, but these usually need addressing also, as described later in this chapter.

SOCIAL COMORBIDITY

Identification of social issues is essential to working with any person with schizophrenia (see Chapter 5). Appropriate social management of these areas through a problem-solving approach (see Table 13.1) allows cognitive therapy to be used. But if a person is about to be made homeless or is hopelessly in debt, it will be very difficult to engage him or her in effective consideration of the psychotic symptoms. Conversely, if the service is helping him or her with these issues, this can be a major factor in the person's engagement in cognitive therapy, and as discussed in Chapter 6, combining case management and therapy can be synergistic.

The therapist will therefore need to integrate therapy with management of a variety of comorbid social problems, including:

- Unemployment
- Social isolation
- Relationship problems
- Parenting difficulties
- Poor living conditions
- Poor social and domestic skills

Treatment for schizophrenia has to be in the context of adequate case management where—as is usual—such social issues exist.

PHYSICAL COMORBIDITY

Therapists will also need to gauge the impact of physical illnesses when these are present or the person is likely to be at increased risk because of the consequences of his or her social and psychological problems (e.g., respiratory illnesses from smoking and diabetes from obesity). Ill-health and death rates for people with schizophrenia are markedly elevated, and assistance with developing healthier living styles is important. Exercise, diet, smoking, and the detection and management of early signs of illness through attendance at health screenings and presenting themselves to health services for investigation can all be approached with clients, using the collaborative approach that has been described. Beliefs about diet and exercise or the like can be explored and motivational issues identified and discussed.

Long-standing physical disabilities can be relevant to formulating a person's problems as they relate to potential causes and the impact the disability has on their lives,

TABLE 13.1. **Problem-Solving Stages**

- Clarification and definition of problems
- Choice of achievable goals
- Generation of solutions
- Choice of preferred solutions
- Implementation of preferred solutions
- Evaluation

Note. After Gath and Mynors-Wallis (1997).

especially in terms of vulnerability and social contact. Physical symptoms from ill-nesses and disabilities can be delusionally misinterpreted—for example, as punish-ment. Impairment of sight and hearing has also been demonstrated to constitute a vul-nerability to psychosis, possibly through interference with the ability to "reality test" and the increased distortion of perception, which in turn can cause confusion and dis-tress. These impairments and disabilities are also stressors in their own right.

SUBSTANCE MISUSE

There are some general principles covering both alcohol and drug misuse and some distinctions between them. Alcohol and cannabis, in particular, are commonly available drugs that are used by millions of people to relax and as an aid to socialization. Yet, the first is legally available and the latter, in most countries, is not. Cannabis has also been in widespread use in most countries for a much shorter period, and generational differ-ences exist in its use. Its effects, short- and long-term, are less well understood, and some controversy about these still exists.

Amphetamines, cocaine, ecstasy, LSD, and heroin are less widely used, although increasingly common. Heroin seems to complicate the picture rarely—that is, it seems to be a complicating comorbid factor infrequently; however, significant numbers of people presenting with psychosis have used amphetamines and, to a lesser extent, co-caine, ecstasy, and LSD. The role of these drugs in precipitating persistent psychotic ill-ness is not yet fully established, but they certainly produce transient psychotic states. Many people who develop persistent illness after the use of these hallucinogenics seem to experience persistent symptoms that closely resemble—may even be identical to—those that they experienced in their first drug-induced psychotic illness. Whether this "caused" the continuing problems hardly matters in practice with that individual. What is important to establish is what the current effect of use of illicit drugs might be. It may also be therapeutic to work on reattribution of current symptoms back to the original drug-induced psychotic episode.

Most cognitive therapy studies in this area have included people using illicit drugs but have excluded those who are using sufficient amounts to warrant a primary diag-nosis of dependence on substance misuse. This means that issues having to do with the use of drugs have featured commonly, but high levels of usage have not. There is still relatively little work on the latter with the exception of one published study (Barrowclough et al., 2001; therapy described in Graham et al., 2002).

Any client using illicit drugs is likely to be concerned about the therapist's attitude toward him or her—specifically, that it will be judgmental and possibly punitive. It is reasonable to normalize the experience without justifying it—for example:

"It is true that many people do take illicit drugs and seem to have few negative ef-fects. Unfortunately, you seem to have been particularly vulnerable to their nega-tive effects."

It does seem that some people are particularly vulnerable—whether biologically deter-mined or, rather a function of their circumstances at the time that made them suscepti-ble to negative effects. For example, they may have recently been in trouble with the police for some reason and were already anxious about using drugs—for example, a friend gets arrested at the same time, and they fear that they will be falsely accused of informing to the police about them or—even more frightening—the drug dealer and his associates. This may well make any negative effects, fear, paranoia, or hallucinations worse and more persistent. It is quite possible then that minor triggers may bring on symptoms—for example, small amounts of illicit drugs, smelling someone else smoking cannabis, or a TV program about drug dealers that they might conceive as referring to themselves.

The management of comorbid drug and alcohol misuse begins with assessing the degree of effect, both positive and negative, that the substance is having. Specific measures to deal with the substance misuse will be needed whenever it interferes with functioning through:

- Repeated precipitation of psychotic episodes that follow directly from and relate clearly to substance misuse.
- Perpetuation of symptoms with the continuing use of substances.
- Social disruption—for example, financial problems, relationship problems, or the loss of or the likelihood of the loss of one's accommodations.

Such remedial measures have tended to focus on minimizing the harm caused by the substances through a motivational interviewing approach preceding the symptom work for psychosis described in this manual. This involves drawing out the risks and benefits of continued substance misuse with the person and then collaboratively negotiating a way of progressing. Dealing with the substance misuse as the priority issue makes sense when someone is unable to participate in any therapeutic work because of:

- The direct effects of intoxication on attention, motivation, and concentration.
- Distraction by concern about where the next drink or drug is coming from.
- The need to resort to substances when difficult issues rise—although the pace of working with cognitive therapy in psychosis can reduce this as an issue.

In cases where the substance misuse has been a coping strategy for managing voices or other symptoms, it can be helpful to outline how specific work may help alleviate the distress the client is experiencing—as an alternative and much more effective and lasting remedy in the long term. However, you may have to agree that substances work quicker and even more reliably in the short term. Instilling hope of a better future is important here, as elsewhere, and despite substance misuse, sometimes a "taste" of what is possible can be beneficial to engagement—for example, some brief work on coping strategies.

The effect of substance misuse on others needs to be considered. Caregivers and staff can be supportive, collusive, or, alternatively, can have very mixed and unhelpful, albeit understandable, attitudes and reactions. It may be difficult for them to be objective about substance misuse. As was noted earlier, for some people, including those with psychoses, alcohol and drugs may not be psychologically harmful, and dogmatic attitudes may interfere with their treatment. An all-or-nothing attitude on the part of caregivers and staff can lead to needless confrontation, angry outbursts, and the precipitation of psychosis. Helping care providers to step back and not make a difficult situation worse requires great tact and diplomacy. Such caregivers should be assured that their overall goals are right, that is, that the person cared for should get better, should have less severe and distressing symptoms, and, ideally, should misuse substances less. But prohibitionist tactics simply do not work: it is far more likely that the person will misuse substances if they constantly encounter arguments about it. Permitting freedom of action allows the person the opportunity to take responsibility for his or her own drug problem—and that includes not blaming caregivers for the consequences of substance misuse. Clients rarely need to be reminded about the concerns that caregivers have—so education of that sort is not needed—but taking a negotiating approach with the client caregivers when called on to provide support can be successful. Collaborative work with caregiver expressed emotion fits well in this context.

Often concerns are expressed about what will happen if illicit substances are combined with medication. These concerns can be straightforwardly answered. A combined sedative effect is a key outcome in most circumstances, but this needs to be considered dependent on the precise medication regime. Also, caregivers may wish to ban visits with friends who also misuse substances,—which can be major problem if the person's only friends fall into this category. Restricting access to friends is, on balance, counterproductive, but shaping alternatives whenever available may be a more successful way of managing this situation. Control of finances is another area where conflict can arise. Indulgence by caregivers occurs when they financially support a person's drug habit, usually for unclear and often conflicting reasons. After collaborative consultation, this practice should be discouraged, although a fear of the consequences may make this decision difficult. However, the client determines the use of his or her own money, although the decision may be subject to other people's influence.

In sum, alcohol and substance misuse are factors contributing to risk of harm to self and others, so their importance cannot be underestimated; but a balanced collaborative approach is most likely to be successful in managing them.

PERSONALITY DISORDERS

It is probable that anybody can develop psychotic symptoms. Whatever personality type presents will shape the clinical picture that emerges. However, whenever that person has serious long-standing and enduring patterns of behavior that cause difficulties in relationships, this will complicate presentation and can do so in a variety of ways. In general terms, the evidence of effectiveness of interventions with most personality disorders is limited—it is even more limited where it is complicated by psychosis. But in practice the most complex cases are those with such a diagnosis (often complicated further by substance misuse).

The types of personality disorder most commonly presenting are borderline, antisocial, schizoid, paranoid, and dependent personality disorders.

Borderline Personality Disorder

Many people with borderline personality disorder (BPD) present with flashbacks and auditory hallucinations that cause distress, as well as diagnostic difficulties. Conversely, there are a significant number of people meeting the criteria for schizophrenia or schizoaffective disorder who have borderline characteristics. It is pointless to get into an argument as to whether these people have one diagnosis or the other. They may well move from one to the other. Indeed, if therapy is effective for psychosis in enabling them to reattribute "voices" to being internal rather than external phenomena, the BPD becomes the major focus of further work and the "psychotic" symptoms become better understood and recede. It is at this point that the work described in Chapter 10 on hallucinations can become pertinent; such work focuses the negative content of voices, which frequently mirrors the beliefs about themselves that have been inculcated in them through previous abusive experiences.

Many practitioners working with BPD exclude those with psychotic symptoms. This exclusion seems unfortunate, as work on the psychotic symptoms themselves is often relatively straightforward in terms of reattribution, as described above. Work on the psychotic symptoms enables work on the issues relating to BPD. Our experience and that of others working with this group is that, once that reattribution has occurred, the client becomes increasingly resistant to reversion to previous psychotic beliefs about the voices. It may be that dealing with past traumatic events needs to be more through understanding the implications and beliefs than by concentrating on exposure to the events themselves, but such a modification to usual practice can be successfully undertaken. It is probably true that those with psychotic symptoms are more severely disturbed—but not necessarily. We have certainly seen people with BPD and very severe psychotic symptoms make good recoveries with a combination of approaches used in a flexible manner. This may mean that the people concerned cannot attend the usual group settings and complete the same exercises that dialectical behavior therapy advocates but that much of the essence of such programs can be utilized on an individualized basis.

Antisocial Personality Disorder

Many people who present with antisocial personality disorder (APD) and psychosis do so in the context of substance misuse that precipitates psychotic episodes. This is compounded by increasing paranoia and often impulsivity that manifests itself toward themselves and others. This may be through physical harm to self or others. Management of psychosis can be disrupted by difficulties in collaboration over medication and social and psychological therapy. Such cases therefore present some of the most difficult challenges. Such clients often come into services because they have been convicted of criminal behavior, or are trying to avoid such conviction, and may require management in secure services. In cases where substance misuse is an additional issue, the constraints of secure hospitalization may eliminate such misuse—short-term—although if on "open" wards, this can be a persistent problem. In the latter instance, however, work on substance misuse issues, as described above, may be quite possible. Medication in hospital settings under involuntary treatment provisions can also be given reliably—and often successfully in terms of managing psychotic symptoms. This can also be a time when therapeutic work on the links between the initial symptom development and those which led to presentation can be focused on.

What often then remains is management of the impulsive and antisocial behavior, including noncollaboration with treatment, and a possible return to substance misuse as limitations on personal freedom are progressively lifted. Management of the psychosis may not be as difficult as that of the substance misuse and personality issues, but it does complicate it. Confrontation and challenge to impulsive behavior may lead to increased agitation and thus precipitating psychotic symptoms, including paranoia and thought disorder. Yet, it may be very important to work at modifying behavior by ensuring that misbehavior does not occur without consequences—that is, that clear unambiguous limits are set. Consistent management from staff and caregivers can be difficult to achieve but over time can be effective. At times this may involve sanctions, including the involvement of police, but careful management calibrated against the ability of the person's psychotic state to cope with confrontation of antisocial behavior is possible.

Other Personality Disorders

All other personality disorders can occur, further complicating psychoses—at least in theory. People with dependent personalities can sometimes prove significant problems diagnostically, in distinguishing them from those presenting with psychoses with predominant negative symptoms. Dependency, however, tends to be a longer-term problem than psychosis—emerging during childhood and early adolescence, when psychosis is rare. But dependency with psychosis can occur, and assisting the person in taking responsibility for his or her actions can complicate the management of negative symptoms, where generally the aim is to reduce pressure. Graduated assistance in beginning to take on roles and responsibilities still needs to be carefully handled, but it may be that some insistence can become appropriate in these circumstances.

People with schizoid ("isolated, withdrawn") and paranoid personalities also present diagnostic difficulties, although again being sure about the client's behavior prior to illness and especially during his or her early years can clarify this. However, where psychosis coincides with these characteristics, it may not be realistic to strive for social integration to any significant degree, although the person's own wishes will guide this.

OTHER MENTAL DISORDERS

Any mental disorder can coincide with psychotic illness and merge with it. For example, many people with voices go through a period of *obsessional rumination* as they recognize that their voices are internal phenomena (see Chapter 1). Indeed, the sole difference between obsessions and voices may be that the former are recognized as egosyntonic whereas the latter are ego-alien (i.e., believed to be internal as opposed to external). Content may be identical. With some people this obsessionality can become a more appropriate focus of therapeutic intervention than the psychosis; for example, one person was obsessed with the belief that her nose was big, another that she smelled, and another that people would think she was gay. The ruminations about these beliefs were much more resistant to treatment than the psychotic symptoms as such and required concerted cognitive behavioral work.

Anxiety frequently coexists, and management is as necessary as in cases where it does not—indeed, it can positively influence management of psychotic symptoms, possibly interrupting their development or elaboration. Therapy can generally take the form of anxiety management used in those without psychotic symptoms. There has been concern that relaxation exercises and/or meditation might precipitate psychosis because of introversion and contemplation leading to decompensation, but this has certainly not been our experience—indeed, colleagues are developing the use of "mindfulness" for management of voices. Of course, if the person finds it uncomfortable or it increases symptoms, especially voices, it is wrong to expect him or her to persist with such discomfort.

Depression is a very common accompaniment and needs management in its own right—it may be consequent to distressing symptoms or may sometimes precipitate them. For example, depressive symptoms may include psychotic ones—delusions of reference, worthlessness, nihilism and bodily change, paranoia, and hallucinations. If these persist, particularly after the mood has improved, a diagnosis of schizoaffective disorder—even schizophrenia—may be made. Suicidal thoughts may become hallucinations by reattribution to other sources ("I couldn't possibly think something as terrible as to take my own life"), which seems particularly common where prohibitions on such actions exist, for example, religious prohibitions or simply because of the responsibilities of parenting or other caring ("I couldn't think such a thing—what would happen to my children/"). This may particularly occur subsequent to or coincident with puerperal depression.

FORMULATION AND COMORBIDITY

A formulation-based approach is central to the management of comorbidity. It enables:

- The understanding of individual symptoms such as, for example, the factors relating to substance misuse. This may directly relate to psychosis (e.g., the use of alcohol to reduce anxiety and, at least in the short term, reduce intensity of voices) or be incidental to it, either preceding it or accompanying it.
- Goal-selection that is appropriate and realistic (e.g., managing social phobic symptoms may need to follow exploration of delusions of reference).
- Selection of appropriate techniques (e.g., exposure work with posttraumatic stress disorder may activate positive psychotic symptoms if not graduated sensitively).
- Coworking with other therapists and agencies, where they are involved, coordinating responsibilities.

Relationships between the person's various symptoms, problems, and comorbid conditions will be drawn out by formulating the assessment of the person's background, situation, and needs into a coherent picture. People with psychosis need treatment for other distressing and disabling conditions as much as, and generally in the same way as, anyone else. The major difference seems to be that their tolerance of heightened emotion may be less—as they can become more psychotic—so treatments that are anxiety-provoking may need more caution. However, more cognitively based approaches can be successful—for example, looking at thoughts about experiences rather than getting the person to reexperience them in real time or in their imagination.

COMORBID CONDITIONS

Gordon (*sensitivity psychosis*): Depression and anxiety, especially in social situations, were relevant to Gordon. Management of depression was along medical lines, with antidepressants and a brief review of the issues that were relevant—particularly the psychotic symptoms and the situation he found himself in. Work on psychotic symptoms therefore predominated. His social anxiety, though present, did not require direct work, although some individual social skills training was relevant and used with him. The beliefs about thought broadcasting and delusions of reference were related to the social anxiety, and as work progressed with them these associations were discussed as having some explanatory value for the psychotic symptoms.

Craig (*drug-related psychosis*): Drug misuse has been a key problem for Craig and precipitated his illness. Relating current symptoms to this initial episode has proved valuable in understanding the phenomena and reattributing the psychotic experiences. His use of substances has gradually discontinued, although this was complicated by his lack of friends who were not using cannabis and speed themselves. He has discontinued seeing the ones who were users, but this has led to isolation, which now is being addressed by his care manager.

Gillian (*traumatic psychosis*): Issues of substance misuse did not feature with Gillian, although they can complicate traumatic psychosis. Dependency, depression, and anxiety, however, were major factors and needed individual management.

Paul (*anxiety psychosis*): Again, no issues of substance misuse or personality disorder presented, but depression was an issue impacting on Paul's beliefs and needing management through direct work on the symptoms themselves and with regard to underlying issues of depression and self-esteem.

FOURTEEN

Relapse Prevention and Finishing Therapy

RELAPSE PREVENTION

What is "relapse"? For our purpose, it is most useful to consider it to be a worsening of distress or disability (usually manifested by increasing symptoms or reemergence of symptoms), or a change in the nature of symptoms (e.g., from neutral to negative content). Relapse tends to mean a *significant* worsening in the person's condition or increase in symptoms, but any cutoff point is arbitrary (although it may have its value in measuring outcome in research studies.) From the client's and caregivers' point of view, any worsening is relevant. Relapse can result from fatigue and weariness at coping with symptoms, as well as from changing circumstances or discontinuation of medication.

Relapse prevention is a key aspect of all the work done with symptoms so far. It is based on a formulation that enables the person to understand and come to an acceptance of what has happened to him or her ("integration"). This acceptance is at the other end of a spectrum from denial and avoidance of any reminder of the acute episodes ("sealing over"), which may include avoidance of any form of mental health intervention. In between is the natural response of "wanting to move on" and the reaction to the stigmatizing effect of the term "schizophrenia" or "psychosis." Some denial may even be a helpful reaction (through reduction of distress), provided that it does not blunt responses to emerging issues.

The worsening or reemergence of symptoms has both individual and common features. Most people experience unease, anxiety, or stress (whatever term they use to describe this is useful to identify). The change may be directly related to life events, and a risk can be that the events are so preoccupying clients that they stop looking after themselves and their mental health until they are overwhelmed. Sometimes the relationship to life events may not be clear—either because the stress is low-key but enduring, or because it is of a specific type that triggers specific anxieties to which the person is susceptible. It can be very difficult to identify any specific stress, although after a relapse, most people with schizophrenia can find something relevant; this may be important because of its potential value for preventing future relapses. However, the search for triggering events shouldn't delay dealing with the emergent symptoms. Occasionally, the obsession with finding a cause can be used to avoid taking sensible measures (e.g., medication recommencement or adjustment).

Specific phenomena that trigger relapses may include the following, and patterns may be detected in these:

- Particular times of the year, week, or day
- Meetings with specific people (e.g., father-in-law), especially if they are going to be present for a certain period (e.g., a holiday weekend)
- Anniversaries—of becoming ill, of losses such as bereavements (including significant events in a client's life—birthdays, etc.), or of hospital admissions
- Changes in medication
- Watching a film or a TV program, or listening to music (any of these may be a reminder or trigger in some other way)
- Use of alcohol or drugs (or even use of these substances by others)

A relapse "signature" (an individualized pattern) can include a change in sleep pattern (especially a reduction in amount), tiredness, anxiety and depression, and/or the reemergence of psychotic symptoms. Initially, the psychotic symptoms (e.g., voices) may develop with the person retaining full insight. There may also be an increase in frequency or negative content, olfactory delusions, or delusions of reference or paranoia (Birchwood et al., 1989). "A touch of the schizophrenia's coming on" was how one client described the return of psychotic symptoms. The "fear of going mad" has been described as a frequent initial symptom preceding relapse and so needs to be handled carefully. It is easy to see how a vicious circle of increased anxiety in a client, a caregiver, and even a mental health worker can increase symptoms and lead to the feared outcome. Sometimes just a sense of unease can begin the cycle, or a physical symptom such as pain (e.g., headaches or backaches) may be the start.

The role of caregivers, friends, the family doctor, and others can be pivotal in intercepting relapse. They have often identified early warning signs occurring previously and can discuss these with the client and yourself. This information can assist in defining the relapse signature, and also in identifying when symptoms are emerging. Caregivers and others may sometimes experience understandable anxiety when behavior that preceded previous episodes, but that may not *necessarily* imply relapse, occurs. Assertive or rebellious behavior can particularly fall into this category and may need careful assessment and negotiation. However, usually it turns out that the caregivers or others are right (although sometimes this is a self-fulfilling prophecy, and work for the future may need to center on helping them respond differently to such behavior). Occasionally, though, other people may not be able to identify and articulate exactly what the prodromal signs of relapse are.

Avoiding Relapse

Avoiding relapse is a reasonable aim, but the personal costs of doing this can be considerable. Many people with schizophrenia avoid contact with the world and withdraw into their homes and personalities with this aim, so a balance has to be struck between the risks of relapse and the advantages of living as normal a life as possible (see Chapter 12 on negative symptoms).

Access to supports—including mental health services, friends, family members, and medication—needs to be available, along with a readiness to use such access. Continuing contact with services may make this more likely, even if this contact consists only of an annual appointment to keep in touch, provide an update on progress over the year, and review the next year for any possible stressful events. Sometimes it helps a client just to know that the service is still where it was before (i.e., it hasn't moved, changed its telephone number, or changed personnel). If personnel have changed, a brief introduction can assist in the future.

It is not necessary to wait for a relapse to occur before developing a strategy for managing it. You may be meeting a person for the first time; the client has just been referred to you because he or she has recently moved into your area, or the client's previous worker has just left, or one of the inevitable changes in services has meant that this person has now been allocated to your care. It is understandable to want to avoid any discussion that might precipitate relapse, but this needs to be considered very carefully.

How much do you know about what has happened to the client? How much do you understand the formulation of his or her problems? Has an effective cognitive-behavioral formulation been drawn up with this client? If not, it may involve extra time to develop one with him or her, but the time saved in reducing the likelihood of relapse can be much greater. It also helps the engagement process and increases the likelihood that the client will approach you if he or she has concerns. It probably improves with collaboration with the treatment plan as well. You can ask questions such as these:

"Can I just clarify what's been happening to you?"

"Do you feel you understand it reasonably well yourself?"

If the person doesn't want to talk about what has happened or discuss specific incidents, this wish certainly needs to be respected, but usually people are only too pleased to go over what has happened to them. Quite frequently, when the events leading to and including acute episodes (i.e., the antecedents and experiences) are not discussed, the person is left confused and fearful of future relapse. This confusion and fear then make such relapse more likely. If the person becomes distressed, it may well be that further discussion needs to be deferred until later (or discontinued completely), but it is important to let the person him- or herself decide on this.

Developing a formulation, as described in Chapter 6, can often be done much more simply and easily when the person is in remission. Not only does it help him or her understand what has happened, but it allows the client (or, with his or her permission, you) to explain to others.

Intercepting Relapse

Once signs are identified, perhaps the most important things for both clients themselves and those around them to remember "Don't panic." It is reasonable to expect symptoms to return, because they are the person's way of responding to stress—it doesn't mean inevitable relapse. Some people get depressed if under stress; others because anxious; others work harder; others get physical aches and pains; others hear voices. Once they have recognized the signs, giving themselves a chance to get help if needed, or to take time out, may be successful.

If it is clear that a relapse is beginning or looks likely, a review of medication makes sense, although it may be resisted. However, if the person assumes that such a review inevitably means increase, and this is confirmed each time (however effective or ineffective the increase may be), this can seriously undermine the chances that the person will pursue other sensible strategies in a collaborative way. "Give yourself a chance . . . ease off" will usually be appropriate advice, but not always; a change as well as a reduction in activities needs consideration. It may even be that reconsideration of the perceived stressor may be sufficient to prevent relapse.

Perhaps the most important element in relapse prevention is a client's feeling of control—a sense that stresses can be handled, and that return of symptoms is not a disaster because they have been overcome before. A sense of empowerment can be fostered, so that use is promptly made of coping strategies. Assertiveness can then be a powerful factor in overcoming stresses and sometimes reshaping relationships that are jeopardizing progress.

RELAPSE PREVENTION

Gordon (*sensitivity psychosis*): Relapse, or worsening of positive symptoms, has been an important consideration throughout work with Gordon. As his resilience and coping strategies have developed, his ability to manage stress (e.g., at work) developed likewise. Defining Gordon's relapse signature has been a focus, although in a gradually developing illness without significant exacerbations (as in his case), sometimes this is difficult to do—simply because there have not been any discrete relapses.

Craig (*drug-related psychosis*): In Craig's case, the ongoing work with positive symptoms has meant that relapse prevention has not yet been a focus. As time progresses, drug use or reminders of drug use may be identified with him as a particular precipitant of relapse, and ways of handling this may be explored. His isolation without his drug-using friends is a related issue currently being addressed.

Gillian (*traumatic psychosis*): Supervision for Gillian is likely to be lifelong, to provide necessary support and to allow opportunities to intervene at an early stage in relapse or worsening of symptoms. With assistance, she may be able to increase her abilities to detect early signs of symptoms; brief recurrence of voices may be the first sign.

Paul (*anxiety psychosis*): Increasing anxiety in response to stress, reduced sleep, and the reemergence of beliefs of a similar type to those presenting initially essentially constitute Paul's relapse signature. With integration of his experiences, this knowledge may prove useful.

FINISHING THERAPY

Two general situations arise whereby termination of therapy takes place:

- Planned discharge occurs.
  —The therapist and client decide together to terminate therapy, under one of two conditions:
    ○ With support continuing from a mental health service.
    ○ With discharge from the service.
  —A contract of therapy is funded or determined by other external influences, and at the end of that time, termination has to occur because it is required of the therapist.
- Unplanned discharge happens.
  —The therapist is unable to continue, in one of two situations:
    ○ For an unexpected reason, such as a personal illness.
    ○ With some preparation possible (e.g., the therapist is closing his or her practice or resigning from an agency, clinic, or service).
  —The person him- or herself discontinues therapy, under one of two conditions:
    ○ With support continuing from a mental health service.
    ○ With discharge from the service.

How do you decide when to discharge a person? This will depend on various considerations: How long can you justify to funding agencies, supervising managers, and indeed yourself, continuing to see the person? Discharge may be to other areas of the mental health service, and this may depend on your role within it. For example, if you are employed solely as a cognitive-behavioral therapist, the people you see with schizophrenia or other psychosis are likely to have complex needs, and you are likely to discharge such people back to the support of services. If you are a psychiatrist, a mental health worker, or possibly a therapist in private practice, you may be able to see people with schizophrenia for a longer time, gradually increasing the time between visits until discharge occurs.

In an ideal world, clients themselves initiate the process of discharge in collaboration with their therapists. They themselves recognize that they now have the internal resources and external supports to move on. The internal resources are such that either (1) their symptoms have ceased and they feel confident about detecting and handling any incipient relapse, or seeking support at an early stage and preventing it from progressing; or (2) their symptoms continue but have been stabilized, and they feel that their coping strategies are sufficient for them to get on with life (but that they can make contact if necessary). The use of medication may continue after discharge, but in some circumstances, the person makes a considered decision to discontinue. This choice may influence your decision about collaborating with discharge—as may your interpretation of whether the client has insight or not into the symptoms—but should never in itself be a veto on it. Stability, supports in place, and the person's desire to discontinue therapy are more important determinants. External supports are those particularly involving confiding relationships with friends, family members, and other health and social services, as well as meaningful activity (though not necessarily employment). A person who remains very isolated and guarded about his or her symptoms is probably not ready for discharge—although a few people who have never seemed to need close relationships, and who have built up a lifestyle that is not dependent on others, may be able to survive effectively.

There is a sense in which planning for the ending of therapy (discharge planning) begins at its commencement, so that unexpected events will cause minimal disruption to the person. Each of these situations calls for a different response. Initially we will deal with the first instance, which is the desirable situation. The process of engagement is one that is designed to maintain the person in therapy and reduce the likelihood of premature termination, but the processes involved in cognitive-behavioral therapy—collaboration, feedback, empowerment—are intended to lead to successful termination. Dependence on the therapist may occur early in therapy and be perfectly appropriate, but by the time of termination, an independence and assertiveness should have developed, so that the person as much "discharges the therapist" as vice versa.

With a psychotic illness, it may seem that support and supervision from mental health services will inevitably be continuous. The treatment and support processes are certainly likely to require years rather than months, but we have had a number of clients with schizophrenia who have made a recovery from very severe illness to discharge us. There are many more who have low levels of contact (once or twice a year), on the basis that access to services can be prompt if needed and that relapse prevention is an ongoing process.

Timing of therapy is an important component in discharge planning. In acute illness, meeting a couple of times a week may be desirable for a week or two, but weekly or biweekly sessions seem more comfortable and effective for people with schizophrenia—and economical for therapists. The work done in a session can be considered, reconsidered, and acted upon in the period between sessions. More examples of circumstances causing concern will arise, allowing constructive discussion to occur. However, once active therapy is beginning to decrease, the person may have achieved a degree of understanding of the symptoms and an ability to cope with them, or they may simply be causing less distress and occurring less frequently. Then extending the period between sessions allows for a maintenance period, although often with continuing gains. It also allows time to build up supports for the future. These may be from mental health services; the person may be getting to know a case manager or care coordinator better and developing a good relationship. (Ideally, the therapist can transfer to that person some understanding of the formulation developed, of the techniques being used, and of the relapse prevention strategy.) Assessment of other available supports (family, friends, family doctor, church, social groups), and of the person's capacity to use these supports, is also very important.

Unpredictable events impinging on therapy (e.g., a therapist's departure) need to be prepared for as early as it is known that they seem likely to occur. If therapy is unfinished, transfer to another therapist is ideal, but may not be possible. It may be possible that another worker (or even a family member) not trained in cognitive-behavioral therapy for psychosis can offer some support.

When people discharge themselves, they may be prepared to consider contact at some later specified date. They frequently come back later, but if not, it is important to ensure that those continuing to see them have details of your work, so that they in turn can take advantage of it in their future relationship with the person.

For most people with schizophrenia and their therapists, discharge from therapy is a very positive experience in which it is possible to reflect on the work done and the positive changes seen. Further support may be necessary, but the improved understanding and ability to cope with difficult circumstances and symptoms will remain with them into a much more hopeful and optimistic future.

FINISHING THERAPY

Gordon (*sensitivity psychosis*): The nature of Gordon's symptoms is such that finishing therapy in the broadest sense is a long way off. He will need support as he eases back into work, and then while he is in it and developing relationships. This means that contact on a gradually tapering basis, with increases in frequency when relapse concerns arise, will be needed. Much of this work can be done by trained and supervised case managers, however, and this may be the most appropriate way of working—until he discharges us.

Craig (*drug-related psychosis*): Similarly, Craig's symptoms may need lengthy work, but focused work on specific symptoms based on a formulation is quite possible and may be very effective. Again, case managers will need to work closely with Craig to provide ongoing support.

Gillian (*traumatic psychosis*): Supervision is likely to be needed for Gillian even when her symptoms have resolved because of her underlying vulnerability, but it would certainly be appropriate to discharge her from therapy after the work has been done (with guidance provided to the care manager and Gillian on further use of coping strategies, etc.). Often the termination period can be difficult, and sometimes symptoms return afterward. The support provided by the therapeutic relationship needs to be transferred to others—to continue, realistically, the process of empowering Gillian herself to become more self-reliant.

Paul (*anxiety psychosis*): Once Paul's symptoms are resolved (or, at least, their impact on his life is significantly reduced), finishing therapy can occur collaboratively—perhaps with Paul himself taking the lead. Again, work on avoiding and managing relapse can assist in termination.

FIFTEEN

Difficulties in Therapy

In this manual we have described a variety of ways of developing and implementing formulation-based treatment programs to work with people with a wide range of symptoms. Nevertheless, sometimes situations develop that do not seem initially to fit into the patterns that we have so far described. So, this final chapter outlines key strategies or refers to where appropriate advice exists in this manual for dealing with a number of problem scenarios that you can encounter in therapy:

- Engaging the actively psychotic person who lacks insight.
- Engaging the unmotivated alogical self-neglectful person with schizophrenia.
- Dealing with delusions that are grandiose and systematized.
- Working with new affects (e.g., depression, shame, or guilt) emerging during the process of therapy.
- Working with the risk of aggressive behavior.
- Working with suicidal ideation.
- What to do if the therapist is incorporated into the delusions.
- How to deal with hallucinations occurring within sessions.
- What to do if the therapist feels that progress is completely lacking.
- What to do if relapse occurs.

ENGAGING THE VERY ACTIVELY PSYCHOTIC PERSON WHO LACKS INSIGHT

Studies of early schizophrenia have shown both cognitive therapy *and* supportive counseling to be of similar effect and both to be significantly better than treatment as usual in improving symptoms generally. It does seem, however, that cognitive therapy is better than supportive counseling or treatment as usual for florid hallucinatory states. For the acutely psychotic person who is often completely lacking in insight, psychological treatment would appear to be very important. The key issues here are to provide brief (10- to 15-minute) regular sessions two to three times per week and to initially focus simply on developing a rapport and a trusting relationship, often aided by appropriate use of normalization. The therapist will begin the process of reality testing at a pace dictated by the person. A series of small clear steps is taken in relation to the perceived areas of distress with the focus on clarifying concerns, repetition as necessary, and very simple experiments. Key issues for the case formulation will often be disclosed during these sessions that should be carefully noted for future reference. Information is delivered only about such issues as the ward routine, medication side effects, relaxation training, and how to elicit support if needed. These sessions will often seem to be initially completely dominated by the client if he or she is actively expressing psychotic symptoms. When the client's behavior is particularly thought-disordered, communication can become very difficult, although the techniques described in Chapter 11 may help to bring order out of disorder.

The therapist should gently structure sessions without attempting to do too much therapy work until the person feels in sufficient control and able to trust enough to begin working on areas of distress. A key therapist error in such situations is to try to move on to symptom management before the person is ready. The key advice in such situations is to go slowly, be open and empathic, and let the person lead until trust begins to develop before moving on to reasoning with him or her and developing alternative explanations.

ENGAGING THE UNMOTIVATED ALOGICAL SELF-NEGLECTFUL PERSON WITH SCHIZOPHRENIA

People with symptoms of the "deficit syndrome" (i.e., "core" negative symptoms, primarily alogia and affective flattening—see Chapter 12) have never previously been considered good candidates for psychological treatment. However, with patience, cognitive therapy does seem to have a very clear role for helping this group. Using the processes described in Chapter 4 to engage, all such cases can be formulated given time. To reiterate, it may be that initial sessions simply involve:

- Sitting together in front of the ward TV.
- Walking around the ward with the person.
- Occasionally commenting on things on the TV or happening in the ward.
- Providing some selected brief self-disclosure.
- Where possible, gently seeking out and engaging with the person's interests— for example, a favorite sports team or even family matters.

The cognitive model, based on genetically, biologically, or environmentally determined vulnerability in relation to stressful life events and circumstances, can be used to understand complex histories. These events and circumstances often accumulate or develop during adolescence, leading to the emergence of delusions of reference, paranoid delusions, affective blunting, alogia, reduced motivation, and self-neglect (sensitivity psychosis). Alternatively, they may present following years of institutionalization in hospitals, residential homes, or even at home in the community (other clinical subgroups). This group seldom engages well with group or individual therapies based on personal motivation, and there is a differentially poor response to medication. These persons tend to have positive symptoms such as hallucinations and delusions that are not heavily emotionally invested or systematized. Symptom management, however, cannot begin until the person has "warmed up a little" affectively. Sessions are focused on identification of anxiety or depression and how this links to current issues. No attempt is made to set any behavioral goals early on. The therapist may inquire about interests or hobbies currently or formerly enjoyed. Affect can then be elicited and identified in relation to these and related thoughts elaborated into conversation.

THERAPIST: What is life like in the hostel?

JAMES: Fine (*no affect*).

THERAPIST: What do you do to pass the time?

JAMES: Look at the paper or watch TV (*no affect*).

THERAPIST: What is your favorite program?

JAMES: The soccer is OK (*no affect*).

THERAPIST: Which team do you support?

JAMES: Newcastle United (*no affect*).

THERAPIST: They used to be good, but I hear they are rubbish now!

JAMES: Alan Shearer is good (*some assertion*).

THERAPIST: He is too slow. He certainly won't score in this Saturday's game (*smiles*).

JAMES: I bet he does (*some assertiveness*).

THERAPIST: I will be listening to the match on the radio. Have you got a radio here? How about listening to 5 minutes of the first half and letting me know how Shearer has been playing when I next see you?

JAMES: OK (*no affect*).

Such therapeutic relationships can develop surprisingly quickly, and it becomes possible to begin to work on related positive symptoms such as delusions of reference, with ongoing facilitation of expression of affect and thought. Often this can lead to formulation after the antecedents have been examined, and symptom management can then begin. However, the principle of paradox should be borne in mind in relation to homework assignments—that is, if you assign the person a task well within his or her capacity to accomplish, the person will not often disappoint you.

DEALING WITH DELUSIONS THAT ARE GRANDIOSE AND SYSTEMATIZED

The key principle with grandiose delusions is to use guided discovery to generate a collaborative case formulation and then work with the links to underlying concerns—that is, the underlying schema. (This group of symptoms usually fits the criteria for anxiety psychosis). These delusions, as with delusional memories, rarely respond to peripheral questioning and reality testing. They should be worked with initially to assess and engage with the person and also to help him or her develop a scientific method of examining beliefs, but rarely will they lead to reduced conviction. Such delusions often emerge after a period of delusional moodiness in relation to adverse life events and circumstances with possible schema invalidation (e.g., a demotion at work affecting beliefs about one's self-worth). The development of the case formulation will often allow the focus to shift from the delusional issues to the pertinent prepsychotic life experiences. This allows a variety of cognitions and affects to be identified from this period. A flow chart can then be worked up (see example in Table 15.1).

This formulation often allows key schemas to be modified, but if not then the techniques of inference chaining can be used once a good collaborative relationship has been established. The inductive chronological formulation above might hint at the possibility that an underlying belief exists that he is to blame in some way for his brother's being taken into care. Discussion of how he felt and what he thought about this event might lead to his stating such a concern, but this needs to be elicited voluntarily—not interpreted or even suggested to him. There would however appear to be compensatory beliefs surrounding a drive for achievement and also a belief that certain things are unacceptable and should not be spoken about. Inference chaining in relation to the delusional belief itself is described below.

> THERAPIST: What would it mean to you if it were true that you had been audiotaped in the cross-dressing shop?
>
> JAMES: It would mean that I would be found out.
>
> THERAPIST: What would it mean to you to be found out?
>
> JAMES: I would be shown to be a disgrace to my family.
>
> THERAPIST: Is that the worst thing about all of this.
>
> JAMES: Yes (*tears and sadness*).

Work at this level of underlying concerns can then proceed, addressing the maladaptive schema—indeed, mistaken belief—that "I am to blame" or "I am a disgrace" and also on the compensatory schemas concerning achievement—"I must achieve at all costs"—and that certain things should never be spoken about. In this case the compen-

TABLE 15.1. Inductive Formulation

0–3 years	Informed that his brother was taken into foster care (*anger and tears*)—"no one will talk about it," "a dark family secret."
3–6 years	Believed that his mother and father were not as emotionally supportive of him as he should be toward them; felt rejected.
6–9 years	Father working "all the hours that God sends." Mother—distant.
9–12 years	Worked hard at school, good at soccer.
12–15 years	Tried on articles of women's clothing to intensify his masturbatory experience.
15–18 years	While in high school, engaged in episodic cross-dressing, felt guilty.
18–21 years	Outgoing with exams. Didn't manage to finish his college thesis despite two extensions. Episode of hepatitis. Trying very hard not to cross-dress.
21–24 years	Went to cross-dressing shop and was fully dressed, felt very guilty about it.
24–27 years	Girlfriend left him after finding cross-dressing material on his computer. Later discovered that she was engaged to be married to somebody else.
28 years	Discovered that his brother had just been promoted at work and developed rapidly increasing anxiety, ending in an acute admission to a hospital.

satory schema was worked with first, as this allowed access to the maladaptive schema. The compensatory schema that certain things being too terrible to speak about was worked with, and a variety of techniques were used including the use of the normalizing continuum and examination of the evidence in relation to the issue of cross-dressing. Thereafter work proceeded on the core belief that he is a disgrace or to blame in some way using role play, examining of the evidence, and work with linked images and memories from childhood. Work on underlying beliefs is usually essential in relation to dealing with systematized or grandiose delusions, and such schema-level work has to be based on a mutually agreed-upon formulation. But if the person is resistant or becomes distressed—as elsewhere—withdrawal is safe and necessary. Other ways of approaching the beliefs can be sought through discussion with colleagues and supervisors. Sometimes it is a matter of waiting and maintaining a relationship with the person, working on other issues until they are ready to look at these beliefs again. Not infrequently, the person surprises you—behavior begins to change despite the absence of a direct discussion of what may seem to the therapist to be critically important work.

WORKING WITH NEW AFFECTS EMERGING DURING THE PROCESS OF THERAPY

As delusions that are not entrenched improve during cognitive therapy with explanations, education, reality testing, and with the generation of alternative hypotheses, people often develop emotions such as embarrassment, shame, or amusement. These should be recognized and dealt with sympathetically during the process of therapy. It should be expected that anyone giving up a belief held for some time, perhaps a number of years, would find it a painful business. In practice, as with all strongly held beliefs, change is slow—short of a process like religious conversion, which is rarely seen in therapeutic practice—and psychological adaptations are made as the changes happen. Nonetheless, belief change can be normalized on the basis that people give up beliefs on a daily basis as new evidence becomes apparent. Examples can be given to the person to make this clear.

> THERAPIST: It is tough to realize that it might not have been the aliens who are visiting now that we have found out about that bird's nest.
>
> PATIENT: I feel stupid.
>
> THERAPIST: I used to always vote for the Tory party, but I realized that they were really too selfish, so now I vote for New Labour. It was a difficult change but worth making.
>
> PATIENT: I suppose so.

In relation to delusions that are grandiose or systematized, without care on the part of the therapist the affects that emerge could potentially be much more painful.

> CLIENT: I am not the son of a Mafia godfather, am I? Just the runt of the family—different, hated, and despised.
>
> THERAPIST: You may well have come to that conclusion as a child, but children often get things wrong, don't they? Can we look at the family photograph album?

After looking at the evidence from the family photograph album, the belief that he was the runt of the family was gradually changed. His mood of anger and sadness also altered as he realized that he had jumped to various conclusions during his childhood on the basis of overheard conversations, and that these could have been viewed in a slightly different way. As he got in touch with long ignored relatives, he was able to test these ideas out, and he came to disbelieve that he was different in some way from the rest of his family.

Again, the key principle is not to proceed if the person is becoming distressed and to maintain hope for a better future. Allowing such behavior as socialization to change before making radical transformations in beliefs means that supports are put into place to support and improve self-esteem.

WORKING WITH THE RISK OF AGGRESSIVE BEHAVIOR

Psychotherapists have often discussed whether it is better to enter the first session with no preconceived ideas of the person or whether it is better to have reviewed the notes and spoken to the person's mental health worker in advance. In relation to the spontaneity of the session and engaging the process, it is probably better for the therapist to have no preconceived ideas. However, this issue is outweighed by the need to know of any previous episodes of risk to self or others and of any existing risk assessments. We would therefore always advocate a complete review of the notes and discussion with the person's mental health worker with a particular consideration of the subject of risk before entering session one. Aggression is more common in people with schizophrenia who are abusing substances, that is, those with comorbid substance abuse and those who have acute schizophrenia in terms of the first episode or relapse. Other risky phenomena include command hallucinations, persecutory delusions, and somatic passivity. In any case, where risk is thought to be a prominent feature, risk assessments should be made by the cognitive therapist and discussed with the mental health worker on a regular basis. A high index of suspicion should be maintained in relation to any of the symptoms listed above or in relation to signs of relapse, increased stress, or increasing substance misuse. Coping strategies should be clearly identified and rehearsed in session and continued even when these, over the medium term, act to maintain the symptom until such times as other strategies can safely be evaluated.

The person who is suffering from command hallucinations will often use distraction and safety behaviors, for example, disengaging totally from the situation after a period of attempting to focus on some other stimulus. These are safety-conscious in the short term in that they reduce risk, and so it may be reasonable to advocate them. However, they may have the effect of maintaining the symptoms. Command hallucinations can be worked on within session utilizing the obsessional thought model (see Chapter 1). The techniques arising out of this model suggest that the person with command hallucinations should practice exposure and response prevention in session in imagery and later on in real life in a variety of graded situations. Also, one can work on such linked schemas as "I must control my thoughts," "Only a bad person would have a thought like this," or "Thinking it or hearing it is as bad as doing it." The normalizing approach enables the person to realize that everyone has occasional automatic, obsessional thoughts at times of stress and that these normal obsessional thoughts have similar themes to the voice-hearing experience—that is, sexual, violent, or religious themes. Usually, using a normalizing explanation, the person can begin to realize that others may get anxious about these thoughts but hardly ever carry any of them out. This allows the imagery, role play, and schema-level work to be undertaken in session in order that the command hallucinations are dealt with differently, leading to homework exercises out of the session. Early work should always be done in session in case the person's voices actually become more commanding before gradually settling down. For this reason it may be best not to deal with command hallucinations by rational responding or by trying to use thought suppression, as these really maintain and exacerbate the symptom over the medium term.

Work with command hallucinations concerning harm to others and (where there is previous experience of acting on voices) also to self should not be undertaken by inexperienced therapists or therapists without supervision. Risks of aggression relating to persecutory or religious delusions are often linked to substance misuse, disinhibition and positive actions, environmental cues, or life events. The person with a persecutory delusional system that he is about to be sacrificed may be triggered into taking positive action by, say, a noisy neighbor moving in next door. It is very important to be aware of such cues when working at the schema level beneath the delusional system. A person with a delusional belief that he is the messiah who will initiate Armageddon on New Year's Eve may actually be tipped into taking action, say, by errant reports on current world events—for example, TV reports on increased terrorist activity.

Somatic passivity when encountered usually responds to diary recording of specific incidents linked to elucidation of triggers and linked affects. Generation of normalizing explanations then helps the person to see that many bodily actions are not completely under conscious control. In all instances involving significant risk, continued dialogue with the psychiatrist and mental health worker responsible should be maintained in case other measures—for example, admission to the hospital on a voluntary or involuntary basis—are appropriate. Despite the obvious worries that always pertain, the authors are not aware of any instances where cognitive therapists were assaulted while working with psychotic clients, or even before or after such sessions.

WORKING WITH SUICIDAL IDEATION

The majority of people with schizophrenia have no active suicidal thoughts most of the time, although their lifetime risk is elevated, particularly during the first decade of the illness. There is, however, a distinct subgroup of at least 5–10% of people at any particular point in time who are making plans to end their lives. It is therefore extremely important to inquire about suicidal ideation, or planning, on a regular basis during cognitive therapy and to record any such intentions or proclivities in the therapy notes. Risk factors such as impulsivity, command hallucinations with passivity (that is, commands by voices that the person is convinced they have to act upon), and substance misuse all need to be considered as part of a comprehensive risk assessment.

It is particularly important when insight increases due to alternative explanations of their delusions being accepted to assess suicidality. The person who comes to a realization—especially abruptly—that he has had a "nervous breakdown" described as "schizophrenic" may have an increase in depression with some increase in suicidal ideation due to the very negative associations that surround the label of schizophrenia. People with schizophrenia often have poor quality of life and have experienced many losses. Working with the pros and cons of continuing, what has been a distressing life (from the viewpoint of the actively suicidal person) obviously requires careful handling. In particular, the pros need to be realistically outlined but hope instilled by discussion of the individual's strengths and potentialities, and more broadly, the major advances being made in this area in terms of the development of new medications, social measures, and therapies. There is some evidence that the overall prognosis for schizophrenia is improving: a long-term follow-up study by a well-respected, long-standing community mental health service recently found that 60% of people with schizophrenia had a good clinical outcome after 20 years (Harrison et al., 2001). As more comprehensive services become increasingly available, such positive outcomes can be expected to continue.

Philosophical and religious attitudes toward suicide are often helpful. Christian and other beliefs may protect the sanctity of life, and religious communities are generally supportive. Buddhist ideas about how working through pain can lead the person to become spiritually stronger can be useful for some people. People often consider ending their lives because they believe themselves to be a burden to others, and they feel that their relatives would be better off without them. However, by discussing the deleterious effects their suicide, would have on others who would have difficulty coping with it, persons inclined toward suicidal ideation and planning can often be encouraged to carry on through these difficult periods.

The concept of suicide as a trapdoor has allowed many people to work through long nights of despair and suffering. They always have the option of suicide as a trapdoor, but they don't have to use it at this particular point in time. Reasons for staying alive in such patents will often come down to, for example, the cat that they are feeding or the key friend or relative who is taking an interest and visiting them now and then. If such issues are being noted in relation to cognitive work on the suicidality, it is important to always highlight several of these reasons for staying alive in terms of personal usefulness in case one of these fails for some particular reason.

Also, helping the client to provide rational responses to automatic thoughts of suicidality or hopelessness theme is useful, for example:

"I am a decent person—my girlfriend and aunts still like me."

"Research will find some new medication or treatment at some point soon which might help me better."

"There are still some things left to enjoy—I will enjoy my brother coming over on Sunday."

For each individual a personalized strategy needs to be developed that usually involves conceptual change, and the description of this is then audiotaped and written on two cards in order that the person might work with these concepts. Death by suicide and even suicidal behavior during the course of cognitive therapy is very rare, and there is also some unpublished research evidence from analysis of data from a recent study (Sensky et al., 2000) that cognitive therapy is protective against suicide in schizophrenia. However, where suicidality is increasing, close cooperation with mental health services is very important to ensure the safety of the person, and further cognitive therapy may need to be suspended if it is clearly related—or may be related—to the person's increasing distress.

WHAT TO DO IF THE THERAPIST IS INCORPORATED INTO DELUSIONS

Incorporation of the therapist into the delusions, while relatively rare, can occur with paranoid delusions that are systematized. It sometimes reflects a relationship that is not developing well; for example, the therapist (possibly working as both a case manager and psychiatrist) may be too busy and keeps being interrupted, or sometimes the client's manner seems to "induce" paranoia. Unambiguous warmth and openness rarely seem to cause such beliefs to be held with any conviction, but sometimes underconfidence and a guarded or relatively unresponsive stance can mar the relationship. If you find that incorporation into delusions is occurring at all commonly, it is an issue worth discussing with peers and supervisors to see whether it is possible to change.

However, once present, it may be worth considering two distinct ways of working. It may be that taking a more relaxed "befriending" stance for a period, with relevant self-disclosure about interests and the like, might prove beneficial, although disclosure of personal material that might increase risk would be avoided. Alternatively or subsequently, moving the focus of discussion relatively quickly to the underlying linked schemas—for example, through inference chaining, as described previously (in Chapter 9)—as more superficial work may be less productive while the therapist is incorporated within the delusion. If the therapy continues at the more superficial level of questioning, with linked homework, then there may be the risk of increasing confrontation in such a setting. Working with the linked schema may allow the person and therapist to again collaborate, although if this becomes disturbing to them the session needs to be concluded as amicably as possible, and if sessions continue they should do so at a slow pace, avoiding distressing areas until the person is ready to discuss them again.

If these ways of working are not successful, a change in therapist may be needed. The risk issues need to be carefully assessed, and where specific threats against the therapist are made, these do need to be taken very seriously. Command hallucinations may also be directed at the therapist, and the related risk issues need to be actively considered on the basis of the likelihood of their being acted upon.

HOW TO DEAL WITH HALLUCINATIONS OCCURRING WITHIN SESSIONS

The occurrence of hallucinations within session can be a marvelous opportunity to use a range of techniques. However, it can also be a sign that the person is becoming increasingly distressed by the progress of the sessions, and so it may mean moving the conversation to less distressing material or gradually winding down the session. However, if the person who is actively hallucinating feels able to continue, work can be done within the session to understand the voices better and to collaborate over ways of coping. Also, the client will be able to test firsthand whether or not other people can hear the voices. The location of the voices can be worked on in the session by the therapist and person together, and the possible mechanisms for their origin can also be discussed. The affective and behavioral responses of the person can be clearly noted, and the automatic thoughts linked to these powerful affective responses can be logged and rational responses worked up. A range of coping strategies can also be attempted within the session to see which, if any, are more effective in giving some control over the voice-hearing experience.

Sometimes hallucinations can be too intrusive. What they say may interfere with the flow of conversation—for example, "Tell him to shut up" or "He's lying to you"—but discussion of these statements has an immediacy that can often be successfully worked with, and an alliance with the client can be further advanced.

WHAT TO DO IF THE THERAPIST FEELS THAT PROGRESS IS COMPLETELY LACKING

A sense of a lack of progress is not an infrequent occurrence at the beginning of therapy prior to the stage at which the formulation has started to become clear. The therapist should in the early stages accept that there appears to be little progress but that as trust builds up the formulation may gradually start to be clarified and, from it, strategies for change can be established. Taking ratings at the beginning of therapy—for example, using PSYRATS (see Chapter 5)—can be valuable, as when these are repeated, evidence of subtle but important improvements on some of the aspects of the psychotic experience often emerge. If progress remains very slow, then the best approach is to reconsider the formulation by going back to the prepsychotic period and personal history and going through this again in some detail. Such perpetuating factors as the relationships with current key figures in the person's life may also be very relevant but often well hidden until a careful reassessment is undertaken.

The techniques used in interaction may also need to be reconsidered. Rational responding—reasoning—about delusions has its limitations, although it is important to work through to engage and assess fully. Moving on to work with underlying concerns is essential if the beliefs are not shifting and may be becoming systematized, but this can be difficult. Key issues may become apparent simply by "standing back," listening to the person and his or her caregivers, and enabling the person to identify important nonpsychotic issues in his or her life. It may be that these can be identified from looking at the issues affecting the individual overall—for example, social isolation, difficult family relationships, poor self-esteem—and other mental health staff may help in this assessment. Also inference chaining (see Chapter 9) may enable you to reach these key issues and work with them. With hallucinations, the person may accept that their voices are part of their illness or at least originating from their mind, but they are not diminishing in the distress they cause. Developing ways of empowering the person in relation to them is generally the best route forward, but this may take time. Keeping records with responses to the voices and developing an assertive dialogue with them may assist.

Listening to audio- or videotapes of your own sessions can sometimes allow you to look more dispassionately at the issues being raised. Most importantly, discussing such difficulties during individual and group supervision with others with an interest or—better—expertise in cognitive therapy can often open up ways forward.

WHAT TO DO IF RELAPSE OCCURS

If the early signs of relapse are present and it is impossible to work using behavioral cognitive or schematic approaches to prevent a full relapse and admission to the hospital, it is important that the therapist keep in contact with the person, if at all possible—for example, visiting him or her frequently to maintain continuity through this difficult period. The therapist will have much to contribute (due to the detailed knowledge of the person and the formulation of the person's difficulties) to the actual management of the person within the inpatient unit. They will be able to encourage staff to produce improvement in symptomatology without excessive use of antipsychotic medication by understanding the issues concerning the person and can help to minimize further traumatic experiences arising from the admission and the ward environment. If the client remains in the hospital for any significant length of time, attendance at the ward round or multidisciplinary review when the person is being discussed can be valuable to all, as the therapist will have much to contribute and will greatly enrich the psychological understanding of the case.

FINALLY . . .

We have learned a great deal from colleagues, editors, and most of all, clients in constructing this manual and continue to do so. We hope you have found it useful, that it will assist you in your practice, and that you can share in the development of effective ways of working alongside people when they experience psychotic symptoms.

APPENDIX I
Health of the Nation Rating Scales

ITEMS

1. Overactive, aggressive, disruptive or agitated behavior
2. Non-accidental self-injury
3. Problem drinking or drug-taking
4. Cognitive problems
5. Physical illness or disability problems
6. Problems with hallucinations and delusions
7. Problems with depressed mood
8. Other mental and behavioral problems
9. Problems with relationships
10. Problems with activities of daily living
11. Problems with living conditions
12. Problems with occupation and activities

Each scale is rated as follows:

0. No problem
1. Minor problem requiring no action
2. Mild problem but definitely present
3. Moderately severe problem
4. Severe to very severe problem

Further details (including full glossary) at www.rcpsych.ac.uk/cru/honoscales/index.htm.

From Wing et al. (1996). Reproduced with permission of the Research Unit, Royal College of Psychiatrists.

APPENDIX 2

Psychotic Symptom Rating Scales

A AUDITORY HALLUCINATIONS

1 Frequency

0 Voices not present or present less than once a week.
1 Voices occur for at least once a week.
2 Voices occur at least once a day.
3 Voices occur at least once a hour.
4 Voices occur continuously or almost continuously, i.e., stop for only a few seconds or minutes.

2 Duration

0 Voices not present.
1 Voices last for a few seconds, fleeting voices.
2 Voices last for several minutes.
3 Voices last for at least one hour.
4 Voices last for hours at a time.

3 Location

0 No voices present.
1 Voices sound like they are inside head only.
2 Voices outside the head, but close to ears or head. Voices inside the head may also be present.
3 Voices sound like they are inside or close to ears and outside head away from ears.
4 Voices sound like they are from outside the head only.

4 Loudness

0 Voices not present.
1 Quieter than own voice, whispers.
2 About same loudness as own voice.
3 Louder than own voice.
4 Extremely loud, shouting.

5 Beliefs re-origin of voices

0 Voices not present.
1 Believes voices to be solely internally generated and related to self.
2 Holds < 50% conviction that voices originate from external causes.
3 Holds ~ 50% conviction (but < 100%) that voices originate from external causes.
4 Believes voices are solely due to external causes (100% conviction).

From Haddock et al. (1999). Reproduced with permission of Dr. Gillian Haddock and Cambridge University Press.

6 Amount of negative content of voices

0 No unpleasant content.
1 Occasional unpleasant content (< 10%).
2 Minority of voice content is unpleasant or negative (< 50%).
3 Majority of voice content is unpleasant or negative (> 50%).
4 All of voice content is unpleasant or negative.

7 Degree of negative content

0 Not unpleasant or negative.
1 Some degree of negative content, but not personal comments relating to self or family, e.g., swear words or comments not directed to self, e.g., "the milkman's ugly."
2 Personal verbal abuse, comments on behavior, e.g., "shouldn't do that or say that."
3 Personal verbal abuse relating to self-concept, e.g., "you're lazy, ugly, mad, perverted."
4 Personal threats to self, e.g., threats to harm self or family, extreme instructions or commands to harm self or others.

8 Amount of distress

0 Voices not distressing at all.
1 Voices occasionally distressing, majority not distressing (< 10%).
2 Minority of voices distressing (< 50%).
3 Majority of voices distressing, minority not distressing (~ 50%).
4 Voices always distressing.

9 Intensity of distress

0 Voices not distressing at all.
1 Voices slightly distressing.
2 Voices are distressing to a moderate degree.
3 Voices are very distressing, although subject could feel worse.
4 Voices are extremely distressing, feel the worst he/she could possibly feel.

10 Disruption to life caused by voices

0 No disruption to life, able to maintain social and family relationships (if present).
1 Voices causes minimal amount of disruption to life, e.g., interferes with concentration although able to maintain daytime activity and social and family relationships and be able to maintain independent living without support.
2 Voices cause moderate amount of disruption to life causing some disturbance to daytime activity and/or family or social activities. The patient is not in hospital although may live in supported accommodation or receive additional help with daily living skills.
3 Voices cause severe disruption to life so that hospitalisation is usually necessary. The patient is able to maintain some daily activities, self-care and relationships while in hospital. The patient may also be in supported accommodation but experiencing severe disruption of life in terms of activities, daily living skills and/or relationships.
4 Voices cause complete disruption of daily life requiring hospitalization. The patient is unable to maintain any daily activities and social relationships. Self-care is also severely disrupted.

11 Controllability of voices

0 Subject believes they can have control over the voices and can always bring on or dismiss them at will.
1 Subject believes they can have some control over the voices on the majority of occasions.
2 Subject believes they can have some control over their voices approximately half of the time.
3 Subject believes they can have some control over their voices but only occasionally. The majority of the time the subject experiences voices which are uncontrollable.
4 Subject has no control over when the voices occur and cannot dismiss or bring them on at all.

B DELUSIONS

1 Amount of preoccupation with delusions

0 No delusions, or delusions which the subject thinks about less than once a week.
1 Subject thinks about beliefs at least once a week.
2 Subject thinks about beliefs at least once a day.
3 Subject thinks about beliefs at least once an hour.
4 Subject thinks about delusions continuously or almost continuously.

2 Duration of preoccupation with delusions

0 No delusions.
1 Thoughts about beliefs last for a few seconds, fleeting thoughts.
2 Thoughts about delusions last for several minutes.
3 Thoughts about delusions last for at least 1 hour.
4 Thoughts about delusions usually last for hours at a time.

3 Conviction

0 No conviction at all.
1 Very little conviction in reality of beliefs, < 10%.
2 Some doubts relating to conviction in beliefs, between 10–49%.
3 Conviction in belief is very strong, between 50–99%.
4 Conviction is 100%.

4 Amount of distress

0 Beliefs never cause distress.
1 Beliefs cause distress on the minority of occasions.
2 Beliefs cause distress on < 50% of occasions.
3 Beliefs cause distress on the majority of occasions when they occur between 50–99% of time.
4 Beliefs always cause distress when they occur.

5 Intensity of distress

0 No distress.
1 Beliefs cause slight distress.
2 Beliefs cause moderate distress.
3 Beliefs cause marked distress.
4 Beliefs cause extreme distress, could not be worse.

6 Disruption to life caused by beliefs

0 No disruption to life, able to maintain independent living with no problems in daily living skills. Able to maintain social and family relationships (if present).
1 Beliefs cause minimal amount of disruption to life, e.g., interferes with concentration although able to maintain daytime activity and social and family relationships and be able to maintain independent living without support.
2 Beliefs cause moderate amount of disruption to life causing some disturbance to daytime activity and/or family or social activities. The patient is not in hospital although may live in supported accommodation or receive additional help with daily living skills.
3 Beliefs cause severe disruption to life so that hospitalisation is usually necessary. The patient is able to maintain some daily activities, self-care and relationships while in hospital. The patient may be also be in supported accommodation but experiencing severe disruption of life in terms of activities, daily living skills and/or relationships.
4 Beliefs cause complete disruption of daily life requiring hospitalization. The patient is unable to maintain any daily activities and social relationships. Self-care is also severely disrupted.

APPENDIX 3
Theory of Psychosis Rating Scale

The scale should not be used for initial assessment sessions or later ones immediately prior to termination. Rate a tape of a therapy session accompanied by a written assessment and formulation.

SECTION I

1) Development of Engagement

Scoring

0—Therapist is over or under talkative . . . does not allow the person time to express his thoughts, does not feedback, does not appear warm or appears overly confrontational or colludes with psychotic thought content.

1—Therapist does allow person time to talk but does not feedback or appears affectively over or under involved. Alternatively therapist allows person to take over. Confrontation or collusion shown by tone of voice or questioning style.

2—Therapist asks appropriate questions but pace and depth may be inappropriate or confrontation or collusion is present.

3—Therapist maintains a good collaborative style through most of the session. Some appropriate use of normalizing of distressing experiences occurs and use of guided discovery made.

4—Therapist attempts to engage the person throughout the session with appropriate questioning, no confrontation or collusion and with warmth. Evidence of relevant normalizing and skilled use of guided discovery.

2) Assessment

This should include evidence of identification of:

    a) Key problems
    b) Key symptoms
    c) Antecedents of the initial and subsequent psychotic episodes
    d) Vulnerability factors
    e) Perpetuating factors

Scoring

    0—No evidence of assessment (from this or previous sessions): key problems and symptoms not identified; no exploration of antecedents
    1—Evidence of assessment limited and inadequate: key problems and symptoms inadequately defined: antecedents either not explored or very limited exploration
    2—Evidence of assessment in most of these areas.
    3—Evidence of good collaborative assessment of these areas, including some work on antecedents and other important factors.
    4—Evidence of excellent and continuing assessment covering all key areas, discussed and may be presented back to therapist by person.

3) Formulation

Evidence of its existence and of it being used as the basis for therapy with development of collaboratively designed and agreed treatment plan. This should also form the basis of the agenda for each individual session.

Scoring

    0—No indication that a formulation exists and that treatment follows an agreed plan.
    1—Some evidence of basic formulation and treatment plan but treatment does not logically follow on from this.
    2—Therapist attempts to work to formulation but unable to retain focus upon it, fails to cover identified topics or alternatively is too rigid when key developments occur within session or to allow further assessment to occur.
    3—Formulation and treatment plan are explicit, e.g., in agenda developed during session or in the summary at the end, and effort is being made to work along those lines flexibly.
    4—Formulation and treatment plan explicit and evolving with therapist skilfully using them as the basis and guideline for therapy with feedback being consistently sought.

SECTION 2

Rater should select which of the following areas should be covered and score accordingly.

4) Reattribution of Hallucinations and Delusions

Normalizing and destigmatizing of symptoms and experiences
Reality testing: Gathering evidence for and against and exploring alternative explanations for example by eliciting possible mechanisms

Scoring

0—No indication that any attempt at reattribution is made.
1—Some attempt at this but haphazard—e.g., ill focused with too many targets or too confrontational.
2—Some useful work—erratically sustained or still too directive.
3—Useful work on some symptoms followed through in a cooperative manner.
4—Symptoms identified in formulation and treatment plan followed through. Intervention appropriate for treatment stage with skilful use of technique, collaboration and feedback.

5) Exploration of Underlying Themes

Where resistant to change, exploring underlying themes to delusions and hallucinations (e.g., using inference chaining).
Reviewing negative content in light of past experiences if appropriate.
Dealing with underlying issues such as low self-esteem, social isolation or guilt

Scoring

0—No useful work done and person may be distressed and no effort made to allay this.
1—Work is haphazard and ill focused and causing distress with too few or too many targets or insensitivity.
2—Some useful work done, therapist does not use appropriate CBT techniques.
3—Useful work and some symptoms followed through. Socratic questioning used but overly therapist-led.
4—Themes are explored appropriately and sensitively and focusing/contributing to formulation. Socratic questioning used consistently with inference chaining where appropriate.

6) Working on:

Coping strategies, relapse prevention and social skills
Expectations with regard to future plans, capabilities and relationships
Short- and long-term goals

Scoring

0—Work would be useful but not attempted

1—Some work done but not appropriate or in obvious areas of need, and ill focused.

2—Some useful work carried out, but with limited collaboration and effect.

3—Useful work done in this area, guided by formulation and treatment plan, in a clearly collaborative manner.

4—The most appropriate issues are being addressed, keeping in mind the stage of the therapy and formulation and followed through in a skilful way.

GLOBAL SCORE

How would you rate the clinician overall in this session as a cognitive therapist for people with psychosis?

0	1	2	3	4	5	6
Poor	Barely adequate	Mediocre	Satisfactory	Good	Very good	Excellent

APPENDIX 4
Informational Handouts

WHAT'S THE PROBLEM?

When you are experiencing problems with stress—even if you think it is other people who have the problems, not yourself—it can be helpful to have a way of describing the problem. This leaflet aims to help you do so.

General terms

Depression—feeling low, unhappy, often with poor sleep and appetite, sometimes you can feel useless, hopeless, even guily of doing things wrong (despite others saying you're not to blame). Thoughts of suicide or even harming others can develop and may take the form of voices speaking to you.

Anxiety—feeling stressed, worried, sometimes with physical feelings: heart racing, breathlessness, giddiness, tingling fingers, headaches, indigestion, and feeling sick.

Obsessions—thoughts go round and round in your head, often they don't seem to be reasonable thoughts but they just keep on going however much you try to stop them.

"Voices"—when it sounds like someone is talking to you or about you but you can't work out exactly where the person who seems to be speaking is—they may seem to be in the room with you but you can't see them or outside it (the leaflet "Understanding Voices" may help explain).

Terms for symptoms like these are useful but often these symptoms form patterns which have been described as, for example, generalized anxiety disorder, manic-depression, schizophrenia, but some of these terms have become stigmatized and are not very good descriptions—schizophrenia particularly has been used to describe a very broad group of problems and has attracted very negative attention over the years. New research using different ways of viewing these problems suggests that there may be more appropriate and acceptable descriptions. Four groups have been identified:

Group 1: Sensitivity—related to a particular sensitivity to stressful events or circumstances.

Group 2: Drug-related—where the initial problems seem to have started after a bad experience with drugs like speed, cannabis, LSD, or ecstasy.

Group 3: Anxiety-based—where stress has built up in someone's life and then they believe that they have found the reason for it, but unfortunately others around them don't seem to agree.

Group 4: Trauma-related—"flashbacks" or "voices" can arise which seem to relate to past traumatic events and can cause severe distress.

The term **psychosis** is used in some circumstances where people hear "voices" which they believe come from someone or something outside themselves, or hold strong beliefs which do not seem to be fully explained by the evidence that they produce in support of them. Often these beliefs and voices are understandable but not always easy to explain to others.

Sensitivity psychosis

This group of problems usually involves:
A slow, gradual onset.

- A feeling of being under a lot of pressure but "ground to a standstill."
- Negative symptoms—difficulty motivating self, "numbed" emotions, trouble communicating.
- A range of problems—especially when under stress—that can include paranoia, voices, unusual beliefs, jumbled thinking.

Help focuses on improving tolerance to stress by initially reducing pressure and setting realistic goals (see leaflets "Getting Motivated" and "Understanding What Others Think").

Drug-related psychosis

The problems:

- Often start with an episode of drug use—especially "hallucinogenic drugs," speed (amphetamines), cocaine, ecstasy, LSD.
- Can involve "voices," "flashbacks," strange feelings—which are very like those occurring with the first experience caused by drugs.
- Can be brought back or be worsened by continued drug use, as can something which triggers a memory of it, for example, seeing an old drug-using friend or a TV program about drug dealing.

Relating the experiences to the original drug use and then working directly with the symptoms can help (see leaflets "Understanding Voices" and "Understanding What Others Think").

Anxiety psychosis

This type of problem usually:

- Originates after teenage years, sometimes when 30 or 40 or later.
- Often it follows a period of stress from work, relationships, and the like.
- Involves a strong belief that seems to provide the explanation for what is happening to the person, but that other people have problems believing—this can lead to conflict and distress.

Help can come from understanding these beliefs (see leaflet "Cognitive Therapy of Psychosis").

Traumatic psychosis

Following a traumatic period, or event—although sometimes years later:

- Distressing "voices" start which say very unpleasant things about the person.
- They may seem to be very powerful and may tell the person to do things—again, usually unpleasant or harmful—often to themselves.
- The voice is often recognizable as someone from the past or at least having to do with past events.

Understanding the voices and learning ways to cope and be assertive with them can work to reduce distress. Feelings about the underlying traumatic events also need to be looked at—as often these make things worse.

Terms are useful, but most important is what is done with them. There is evidence that what helps most is:

- Acceptance that treatment (medication and talking) can help.
- Developing an understanding of the voices and beliefs that are important to you.

Cognitive therapy is one way that may help (see leaflet "Cognitive Therapy of Psychosis").

Professor David G. Kingdon
Department of Psychiatry
Royal South Hants Hospital
Southampton, UK
SO17 0YG

E-mail: dgk@soton.ac.uk

Further reading: *Cognitive Therapy of Schizophrenia* by David G. Kingdon and Douglas Turkington (2005). New York: Guilford Press.

COGNITIVE THERAPY OF PSYCHOSIS

Many people find it very helpful to talk with somebody about the way they are feeling when they are depressed, anxious or confused. One way that has been shown to help with depression and anxiety is to talk about the thoughts that go along with the feelings. So when somebody's feeling low, it may be because they are thinking of their mother who has died or something else that has happened to them.

When somebody is confused and worried about things happening in their life, it may also be useful to try to work out what thoughts are relevant. So somebody may be upset because they are con-vinced that they are being followed or persecuted. It can then be worth trying to work out why they think that might be happening.

Cognitive therapy is a way of trying to identify and then understand these thoughts. They may be thoughts that on the surface seem reasonable but the fears have got out of proportion or things have been taken too personally. By weighing up the "pros and cons" of a situation, it can be possible to look at it differently. It may be that there is an

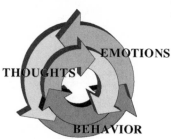

alternative to the conclusion that is causing such distress. Anxiety can cause all sorts of strange feelings like numbness or tingling, pain or breathing problems; these can sometimes be misinterpreted as, for example, electric shocks or physical interference by someone and these concerns may helpfully be discussed.

Sometimes there are beliefs which go back a long way which seem to shape how people view situations. For example, if they grew up to believe they were useless, when something goes wrong they may blame themselves, even if it wasn't their fault. Sometimes thoughts can sound like voices speaking out loud and, when this is happening, cognitive therapy can help people understand and cope with them better.

What Is Cognitive Therapy?

Basically cognitive therapy involves talking to a nurse, doctor, psychologist or other trained person about the concerns and worries and trying to understand them better. This may mean:

- Talking about how problems may have begun
- Discussing how what was happening was interpreted
- Understanding things that happen that seem strange

- Finding out about the sorts of worries the person has

They may be hearing voices when nobody is about, or hear people referring to them as they walk past, or on the TV or radio. There are a variety of other things that can be helped by discussion, e.g., feelings that somebody or some organisation is persecuting the person or knows what they are thinking. On the other hand they may have beliefs about themselves that others don't seem to understand or accept, for example, that they are a particularly special person in some way.

For some people, it may help to:

- Keep a diary of these thoughts
- Identify particular problems
- Find out more about the beliefs and how they might be affecting them
- See if anything particularly makes them better or worse

Coping with troublesome beliefs can be difficult when others don't believe the person. Talking about them with a mental health worker may help them do so.

Can cognitive therapy help with "voices" and strong beliefs?

Sometimes people with psychosis can hear someone, or a number of people, speaking or shouting, but nobody else seems to hear them. "Voices" like these can be very distressing: they may say abusive things about the person or tell them to do unpleasant things. Cognitive therapy can help them understand these voices—that they are usually the person's own thoughts or memories sounding as if they are aloud—and then work out what causes them and what to do about them. Understanding them is important in reducing the fear and anxiety caused and there are also a variety of coping techniques which can help. Strong beliefs can often be understood through reviewing the way stress and vulnerability interact.

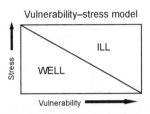

Vulnerability–stress model

What about "negative" symptoms?

When motivation seems very low and the person seems negative about everything, we describe this as having "negative symptoms." There may be a number of reasons for this, sometimes depression, sometimes voices and delusions which are not immediately apparent. Sometimes there is a fear of these symptoms coming back again and so all stress and stimulation is avoided. After an acute episode of illness, a period of convalescence and healing may be needed. Expectations need to be very realistic and sometimes this means a radical re-think; it may be an achievement to just answer a telephone call or watch a TV program even in someone who was previously very capable. Small but readily achievable goals may be set to build confidence. The therapists may even advise that initially enduring a waiting period of just calm stability is appropriate, though not always easy to do. There is now good evidence that cognitive-behavioral therapy helps patients by reducing pressure.

Doesn't it make voices and strong beliefs worse?

There is still a common belief among many doctors and nurses that talking about voices and strong beliefs makes them worse by focusing attention on them. Some psychiatric textbooks have advised against such discussion but there seems no direct evidence to support this. It is clearly wrong to force someone to talk about something if it distresses them but allowing them to talk, as occurs in cognitive therapy, seems humane and can be positive. If the person does become distressed, the conversation can be interrupted and then continue later, if appropriate. Where the discussion becomes repetitive, it probably is sensible to `agree to differ' - a skilled cognitive therapist will then use techniques to overcome such blocks.

Can you use cognitive therapy instead of medication?

All the studies which have shown cognitive therapy to be effective have used it in combination with medication—including using some studies in which clozapine and the newer drugs, like risperidone and olanzapine, have been used. Sometimes people will accept drugs but not cognitive therapy, and sometimes therapy but not drugs—but it seems that the combination is best.

So does it really work?

There is now good evidence from studies in the U.K., Canada, Netherlands, Italy, and Belgium that cognitive therapy helps reduce symptoms. It is used in addition to the usual treatments, can help people understand why, for example, medication is useful so that they are more prepared to take it and help them discuss their needs with their doctor or mental health worker.

How can I get cognitive therapy for my self or my relative?

Initially it is best to discuss this with your current mental health worker or psychiatrist. Because it is so new, there are still only a few trained therapists around the U.S. and many other countries although it is now much more available as part of standard clinical practice in the U.K. Therapists are being trained on `THORN Psychosocial Interventions' and cognitive-behavioral therapy for severe mental illness courses and it is, increasingly, part of basic professional training. Organizations exist in most countries providing information on therapist availability, e.g., Academy of Cognitive Therapy (www.academyofct.org), Association for Advance ment of Behavior Therapy (www.aabt.org), and British Association for Cognitive Psychotherapies (www.babcp.org).

Professor David G. Kingdon
Department of Psychiatry
Royal South Hants Hospital
Southampton, UK
SO17 0YG

E-mail: dgk@soton.ac.uk

Further reading: *Cognitive Therapy of Schizophrenia* by David G. Kingdon and Douglas Turkington (2005). New York: Guilford Press.

UNDERSTANDING VOICES

The information in this leaflet has been useful to a number of people who are troubled by hearing voices. However, some people hear voices and are quite happy with the experience—if you are one of these, the following may not be so relevant to you.

Hearing voices . . .

Hearing voices when nobody is around or at least when nobody seems to be saying the words you hear is quite common. Sometimes the things said seem to come from neighbors, TV, radio, or people you pass in the street. Other times they can just seem to come out of the air.

They seem to be very real; they can be very loud. They may shout at you or sometimes just whisper. They can say all sorts of things. Sometimes the things said are not particularly upsetting, but for most people they are worrying, threatening, or abusive.

They may seem to be talking about you, even telling you what you are doing or thinking. This can be very puzzling, as it is difficult to understand how they can know such personal things. They can be particularly distressing when they are rude or abusive toward you. Sometimes they can swear or tell you to do awful things.

They can sound very convincing as if they have the power to make you do things, even when you don't want to do them.

It can be very difficult to work out where they are coming from. So it may be worth checking whether other people can hear the voices. If they can, they may be able to help you do something about them. Sometimes they can help you work out what or who is saying these things to you.

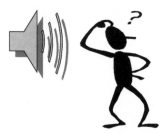

If they can't hear them, you need to work out why that might be the case. It may be that they aren't with you when the voices happen; see if you can tape-record whatever it is you are hearing. Maybe the voices seem to be directed at you alone—only you can hear them. It's worth trying to work out why that might be and talk about it with someone like a nurse, psychologist, spiritual adviser, or doctor who might be able to help. Sometimes it is caused by things happening to you: see the list of "where voices come from."

Voices may seem to be coming from behind you, through the walls, even through loudspeakers. Or it can be very difficult to believe at times, voices that nobody else can hear are sometimes misinterpretations of other sounds or more usually thoughts sounding aloud. That doesn't mean that the voices sound like your own voice; they may be memories of someone else's voice or voices you don't recognize. It may be a man's voice or a woman's voice. Just like in dreams you can hear people speaking, so voices can be thoughts aloud. Memories of other people speaking or of a tune in your head are examples of sounds you can sometimes quite vividly recall.

It is important to understand that voices cannot make you do anything. Thinking that they can't control you might make the voices feel worse initially. But if they are from your mind, it is up to you whether you act on what they say—in other words what you are thinking. But do get support if they seem overwhelming.

There are a variety of ways in which you can lessen the effect of voices or learn to cope with them better.

Where do voices come from?

Voices can occur in lots of different situations:

- When going off to sleep or waking up
- When stopped from going to sleep
- After a bereavement
- Using drugs like speed—amphetamines, ecstasy, LSD, and cocaine
- When you have a very high temperature and with other physical illnesses
- Severe states of deprivation, e.g., in a desert without water
- With illnesses like severe depression or schizophrenia
- When seriously deprived of stimulation, e.g., under conditions of sensory deprivation
- In very stressful circumstances in hostage situations
- Very stressful events like violent attacks, accidents, or intimidation can sometimes imprint themselves on someone's mind as voices

Studies in the United States have shown that 4–5% of the population hears voices at any one time.

What can you do about voices?

The following are methods which have been useful at some time or other to people distressed by voices. Some may not be useful to you, but others may.

- Switch on the radio
- Listen to music (maybe use headphones)
- Have a warm bath
- Talk to a friend
- Go for a walk
- Read a newspaper or magazine
- Make a cup of tea
- Try some vigorous exercise
- Just relax—use whatever method of unwinding that works for you
- Keep a diary so that you can work out when the voices come on and what starts them off; then you might be able to work out ways of dealing with them
- Some people talk about "developing a relationship with their voices" which can help—asking them why they are saying what they say
- Maybe talk with or better ask in your mind why they are distressing you—what right they have to invade your privacy?
- If they say you are bad, see if you can discuss it with them—talking about your good points also
- Some people have found it helpful to allocate a certain time in the day to listen to the voices and then get on with their life at other times
- If they tell you to do something you don't want to do, question them—explain that you don't deserve to be told to do such things and you want to take control of your own life
- Perhaps talk with a doctor about how medication might help with the voices
- Talk with a nurse, doctor, or psychologist about ways of understanding the voices and developing other coping methods

Brain scans of people who hear voices have shown that when the voices are active, there is brain activity in the area that normally indicates that they are speaking. It does therefore seem that voices, at least in the people scanned, is literally "inner speech."

Supernatural or religious voices

The voice can seem like it comes from God or Satan, some supernatural source, or even aliens of some sort. If it does you might want to talk over with someone like a therapist, psychologist, or doctor why you think that that is where it comes from. Has it said that to you itself? Well, is that reason to believe it? Would God say such unpleasant things? Satan (if you believe he exists) might but are you maybe jumping to conclusions that because the things said are so evil that it must be from an evil source like the devil?

Such evil voices can occur as a result of being depressed or the effects of drugs like speed and cocaine. If you do have religious beliefs, you may find additional help through discussion with your spiritual adviser.

Further reading: *Cognitive Therapy of Schizophrenia* by David G. Kingdon and Douglas Turkington (2005). New York: Guilford Press.

Also in some countries, **Hearing Voices Groups** have been set up which can be a rich source of support and information.

Professor David G. Kingdon
Department of Psychiatry
Royal South Hants Hospital
Southampton, UK
SO17 0YG

E-mail: dgk@soton.ac.uk

UNDERSTANDING WHAT OTHERS THINK

Thoughts can sometimes be quite confusing; sometimes this can lead to misunderstandings about the way people communicate or refer to each other. The following might be useful to you if you're feeling confused in this way.

Can you read other people's thoughts or they read yours?

Over the years, many people have tried to work out whether it is possible for one person to read someone else's mind or to get someone to think what the someone else is thinking. In some ways it would be quite convenient not to have to say things and just think them to each other. There have been some instances where twins or brothers or sisters have believed that they have been aware when, for example, the other has had an accident or fallen ill, even when they have been a long way away from each other.

People use the term "telepathy" to describe this and quite a lot of people have some belief that some forms of telepathy occur. Scientists tried to test this in the 1950s and 1960s by using experiments. They got volunteers who would sit in one room and try to transmit a thought to someone in the next room. For example, they would look at a playing card drawn from a pack and the person in the other room would try to imagine which card they were holding. Or a set of cards with shapes or colors on them were used. The results of these experiments were not dramatic—in some cases, it seemed that the guesses were right more often than would be expected by chance but in most the results did not prove that telepathy was possible.

Of course, there are some people who believe that they have a particular ability to read other people's minds, for example, mediums and

some spiritualists. If you ask them to read a particular person's mind, they won't usually do so, so there is not much evidence that they can do what they actually say. Some will be tricksters, others seem to genuinely believe what they say. It is as well to have an open mind but also a reasonable one.

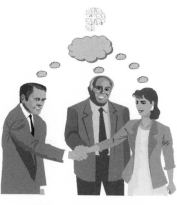

You may feel yourself that you have this power. If you have, does it mean that you think you can read anybody's mind? If so, perhaps it would be worth checking this out with a close relative, friend, therapist, nurse or doctor. Thoughts can work in quite mysterious ways. They are essential to our existence but can sometimes be confusing. Have you ever had the feeling that you know exactly what someone else is thinking? It may be that something they did, which might

have seemed like a sign to you, is the convincing factor.

Perhaps they said something that you are sure they could only know if they read your thoughts. It may just be that you don't feel that you need anything to back up your belief—you just know it to be true.

On the other hand, you might be sure that someone else seems to know just what you have been thinking about. Sometimes it can be embarrassing because the thoughts you had were violent or sexual. Maybe you looked up and saw them watching you and that convinced you.

Try to work out what evidence you have that they can actually know your thoughts. As we said earlier, there is not a lot of evidence to support the belief that people can read each other's thoughts. And there is no evidence that someone can broadcast their thoughts to people around them, even though you can sometimes be absolutely convinced that that is happening. is there evidence that thoughts can be put into your mind or taken out by other people.

Talk with a health worker. See if you can test it out, if you're not convinced. When you are feeling very sensitive, these sorts of beliefs can develop and worry you. They are really an unfortunate diversion from dealing with practical and emotional problems you may have.

How can the TV, music or radio refer to you?

The TV, radio, and music form an important part of most people's lives. They provide relaxation and information but sometimes the things they seem to be saying can seem to become just too personal.

It can seem like the TV presenter, for example, is saying things which must refer to you and you alone. He or she seems to know things about you that are personal and which you may have thought nobody else knew about. They may seem to refer to you by name. It can be very convincing and loud. Certain programs seem particularly likely to cause problems; the news has been shown to be one, but documentaries and programs like *EastEnders* or *Frazier* can also have the same effect.

Words in songs may seem to be directly related to what you are thinking in an uncanny way. It can be hard to believe that they can be intended for anyone but you alone.

When this happens, it can be worth just checking with someone who is with you—if anyone is with you—if they heard anything strange. Perhaps ask, for example, "I thought I heard my name called, did you hear it?"

It is worth noting down what times of day and which programs seem to be related to the problem, or note what is said about you, or what is being said as part of the song. If it is a song or you've got a video of the program, going over it with a therapist, nurse, doctor, or somebody you get on with, may help you work out what is happening.

Of course, sometimes people are referred to on TV, etc., when they've done something that is newsworthy but it is also possible that thoughts may have got muddled, things misheard, or voices caused the problem. If voices might be the problem, you might want to look at

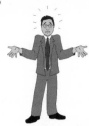

"Understanding Voices," another leaflet in this series.

Having constant references to you can be very disconcerting, particularly when the references are critical or abusive, as they often seem to be. When you have been under pressure or depressed, you can be very sensitive to things happening and this can be very confusing. It can mean you can be oversensitive. After all, why should people on the TV or radio refer to you? What could you possibly have done that could deserve that? It can help to talk these fears and concerns out with other people. Although it is best to talk about them to people who can help, they might just puzzle strangers. is worth working out what may help.

And strangers?

When you are walking in the street or any public place, sometimes it can seem that people are talking about you or laughing at you. This can be very upsetting and worrying and even stop you from going out. Because they look at you and then talk or laugh, it may seem reasonable to assume that they are referring to you. But they may just be thinking about other things—why is it that you think they are referring to you? If you were dressed or behaving strangely, they might, but if not, why? When you are feeling stressed, you can be very sensitive—oversensitive—and sometimes these beliefs can develop out of that.

Coping with ideas of reference or thought broadcasting

- Keep a diary to note when it happens (your therapist can give you one)
- Discuss your diary with your family, good friend or health worker
- Unless it is too distressing or your health worker suggests it, don't stop watching TV, or going out, etc. This just limits your life.
- Why should it or they refer to you? Talk to your health worker, family or good friends about any possible reasons
- Medication may help; talk with a doctor about it

Research about thought broadcasting and reference

The feeling that you are being referred to when that is not taking place is quite common. But when it becomes a fixed belief that doesn't seem to be based on good evidence, it can be distressing and seriously interfere with living. Cognitive-behavioral therapy uses discussion of such beliefs to understand them better and perhaps put them into context so that things are not, inappropriately, taken personally. The information in this leaflet has been carefully researched and results of randomized controlled studies in "treatment-resistant schizophrenia" have recently been published showing the effectiveness of cognitive-behavioral techniques.

Professor David G. Kingdon
Department of Psychiatry
Royal South Hants Hospital
Southampton, UK
SO17 0YG

E-mail: dgk@soton.ac.uk

Further reading: *Cognitive Therapy of Schizophrenia* by David G. Kingdon and Douglas Turkington (2005). New York: Guilford Press.

GETTING MOTIVATED

Has your "get up and go" got up and gone?

Problems to do with stress and mental health problems can seriously affect what we do and how we do it. All areas of life can be influenced—work and study can be difficult to pursue when you feel distracted, have poor concentration, lack the will to do things, or just feel completely exhausted.

While this happens to everybody at some time in their life, when it becomes a persistent problem going on for weeks or months, simply hoping it will get better isn't good enough.

Relationships can be affected because you don't feel like talking or just can't seem to get the words out. It may be difficult to feel close to others when you're distressed or just numbed.

Interests in hobbies, sports, TV, music, going out, friends, and other people may be affected and lead to a decrease in activities This can mean getting increasingly isolated and even if you used

Achieving expectations

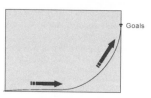

to be reasonably sociable, you can get quite cut off and become socially withdrawn.

Sometimes this can make life feel easier—less stressful—but in the long term can become dull, boring, and depressing.

These symptoms are sometimes called "negative" symptoms (see next page) and can be very disabling. It is very important initially to reduce feelings of stress and then start to set goals, which are well within your capacity to do, with your mental health worker.

Setting reasonable goals

How much time do you need to rest and recover? . . . . months/years

Once feeling more relaxed, what would be your first step to getting back to "normal?"

. . . .

. . . . (Don't complete until you feel ready to do so).

What are your longer-term goals, in 5–10 years' time?

Work/study . . . .

Relationships . . . .

Hobbies/leisure . . . .

Living arrangements . . . .

What are negative symptoms?

The term "negative" symptoms is used to describe a set of problems which are quite disabling and often difficult to understand—in a sense, they are the opposite to "positive symptoms," voices, and strong beliefs—but positive symptoms can lead to negative effects, so they can involve a mixture of causes, including effects of the illness itself, side effects of medication, and depression. They are described by the following technical terms—with a simpler explanation to help you understand them:

Affective flattening: The person may appear to have difficulty communicating emotion or expressing his or her feelings through facial expression. It may be biological in origin or caused by circumstances. It may be that the person is effectively "in shock." This may be related to past traumatic events, e.g., bereavement, or it may be appropriate behavior for the circumstances in which they lived, e.g., if shows of emotion are disapproved of in their family. It may be a direct reaction to abusive, unpleasant voices or thoughts and the "frozen" expression, a "front" to the world, an attempt to cope with seemingly overwhelming disturbance. Depression itself will present with affective flattening. Medication can also contribute. Side effects, e.g., stiffness and reduction in movements of face and body, can be caused by antipsychotic drugs, especially the older "typical" drugs.

Alogia: This can be thought of as `lack of thoughts' but may be difficulty communicating them. One reaction to criticism, real or anticipated, can be to "shut up." Anxiety and perception of pressure certainly can impede communication, causing interruption, even stopping, of thoughts ("thought block").

Avolition: Absence of drive and motivation is possibly the most disabling of negative symptoms. It is certainly one of the most frustrating. The person seems "lazy," "bone-idle," and "never going to get anywhere in life," but perhaps a better expression is "driven to a standstill." Very often it emerges that lack of effort may now seem the problem but this has certainly not always been the case. People with a range of abilities and achievements may present with avolition. A drop-off in performance is common and will often follow failure to achieve expected results and then pressure and anxiety surrounding this. A vicious circle develops where the more they try, the less able they are to complete tasks successfully so the more frustrated and demoralized they become. Others around them may unintentionally contribute by encouragement, which can itself seem to be pressure. Society may also increase pressures, e.g., to get a spouse, job, and family. For many persons this is not an unreasonable long-term goal but a short-term nightmare (see ways of combating on page 1).

Anhedonia: This can be confused with depression but essentially involves a sense of emptiness and so is considered a negative rather than a primarily emotional symptom. It may be related to demoralization, hopelessness, or feeling numbed by stress.

Attention deficit: There is good evidence for poor attention and concentration with mental health problems. Persons do worse on psychometric testing than normal controls. But preoccupation and distraction also occur because of hallucinations, especially when these are vivid and intrusive, but also other thoughts, either delusional, obsessional, or simply very worrying or even interesting to the person. If you think the police are coming to get you or the world is ending soon, it's quite likely that your mind will be preoccupied with that rather than therapy, assessment, or even psychological testing. Overstimulation may also contribute and increase attentional deficit—the more the person tries to attend, the more these thoughts about thoughts ("God, aren't I useless") may interfere.

Social withdrawal: Withdrawal may be an appropriate way to cope with overstimulation, which has long been recognized as an issue in rehabilitation. Social overstimulation may be a particularly unpleasant source of stress.

What can help?

There is now good evidence from studies in the U.K. and Canada that cognitive therapy helps reduce negative as well as positive symptoms. It is used in addition to the usual treatments and can also help people understand why, for example, medication may be useful so that they are more prepared to take it—and discuss their needs with their doctor or mental health worker. Medication can help by reducing positive symptoms—voices, thought disorders, and the adverse effects of strong beliefs—with beneficial effects on motivation and distress. It can also help with depression and some medications-clozapine is the best example—seem to have a direct effect on negative symptoms themselves.

Professor David G. Kingdon
Department of Psychiatry
Royal South Hants Hospital
Southampton, UK
SO17 0YG

E-mail: dgk@soton.ac.uk

Further reading: *Cognitive Therapy of Schizophrenia* by David G. Kingdon and Douglas Turkington (2005). New York: Guilford Press.

APPENDIX 5
Formulation Sheet and Diaries

APPENDIX 5.1. Making Sense

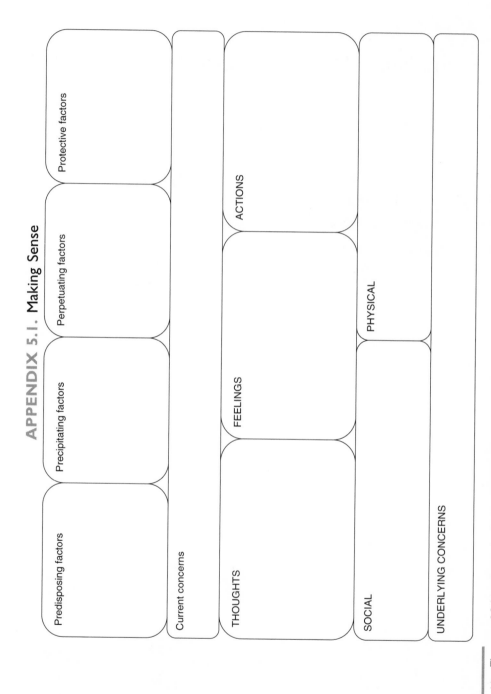

| Predisposing factors | Precipitating factors | Perpetuating factors | Protective factors |

Current concerns

| THOUGHTS | FEELINGS | ACTIONS |

| SOCIAL | PHYSICAL |

UNDERLYING CONCERNS

APPENDIX 5.2. Diary of References

If you think someone is referring to you or talking about you—perhaps in the street or on TV or radio—fill in below what happened.

Date/time	Who did you think referred to you?	What did he or she say?	What do you think it meant?	Is there anything else it could have meant? Why should he or she refer to you?

APPENDIX 5.3. Diary of Thought Broadcasting

If there is an occasion when you think someone knows what you're thinking, fill in below what happened.

Date/ time	Who seemed to read your thoughts?	What were you thinking?	What made you think that they'd read your thoughts?	Were there any other possible explanations?

APPENDIX 5.4. Diary of Voices or Visions

When your voices or visions come back or get worse, fill in below what happened. It may help us understand them better.

Date/time	What did the voice or vision say?	Or what was the voice or vision of? What were you doing at the time?	What did you do in response to the voice or vision?	Was there anything else you could have done?

References

Alanen, Y., Lehtinen, K., Rakkolainen V., et al. (1991) Need-adapted treatment of new schizophrenic patients: Experiences and results of the Turku Project. *Acta Psychiatrica Scandinavica*, *83*, 363–372

American Psychiatric Association. (2000). *Diagnostic and statistical manual of mental disorders* (4th ed., text rev.). Washington, DC: Author.

Andreason, N. C. (1981). *Scale for the assessment of negative symptoms.* Iowa City: University of Iowa.

Asberg, M., Montgomery, S. A., Perris, C., et al. (1978) The comprehensive psychopathological rating scale. *Acta Psychiatrica Scandinavica, 271*(Suppl.), 5–27.

Barrowclough, C., Haddock, G., Tarrier, N., et al. (2001). Randomized controlled trial of motivational interviewing, cognitive behavior therapy, and family intervention for patients with comorbid schizophrenia and substance use disorders. *American Journal of Psychiatry, 158*, 1706–1713.

Beck, A. T. (1952). Successful outpatient psychotherapy of a chronic schizophrenic with a delusion based on borrowed guilt. *Psychiatry, 15*, 305–12.

Beck, A. T., Rush, A. J., Shaw, B. F., et al. (1979). *Cognitive therapy of depression.* New York: Guilford Press.

Beck, A. T., & Rector, N. A. (2002) Delusions: A cognitive perspective. *Journal of Cognitive Psychotherapy, 16*(4), 455–468.

Beck, A. T., Ward, C. H., Mendelson, M., et al. (1961). An inventory for measuring depression. *Archives of General Psychiatry, 4*, 561–571.

Bentall, R. P., Jackson, H. F., & Pilgrim, D. (1988). Abandoning the concept of "schizophrenia": Some implications of validity arguments for psychological research into psychotic phenomena. *British Journal of Clinical Psychology, 27*, 303–324.

Bentall, R. P., & Kinderman, P. (1998). Psychological processes and delusional beliefs: Implications for the treatment of paranoid states. In T. Wykes, N. Tarrier, & S. Lewis (Eds.), *Outcome and innovation in the psychological treatment of schizophrenia.* Chichester, UK: Wiley.

Birchwood, M., & Chadwick, P. (1997). The omnipotence of voices: Testing the validity of a cognitive model. *Psychological Medicine, 27*, 1345–1353.

Birchwood, M., & Iqbal, Z. (1998). Depression and suicidal thinking in psychosis: A cognitive approach. In T. Wykes, N. Tarrier, & S. Lewis (Eds.), *Outcome and innovation in psychological treatment of schizophrenia.* Chichester, UK: Wiley.

Birchwood, M., Smith, J., Cochrane, R. W., et al. (1990). The Social Functioning Scale: The development and validation of a new scale of social adjustment for use in family intervention programmes with schizophrenic patients. *British Journal of Psychiatry, 157,* 853–859.

Birchwood, M., Smith, J., & Cochrane, R. (1992). Specific and non-specific effects of an educational intervention for families living with schizophrenia. *British Journal of Psychiatry, 160,* 804–814.

Birchwood, M., Smith, J., Drury, V., et al. (1994). A self-report insight scale for psychosis: reliability, validity, sensitivity to change. *Acta Psychiatrica Scandinavica, 89,* 62–67.

Birchwood, M., Smith, J., MacMillan, F., et al. (1989). Predicting relapse in schizophrenia: The development and implementation of an early signs monitoring system using patients and families as observers. *Psychological Medicine, 19,* 649–656.

Bleuler, E. (1911). *Dementia praecox or the group of schizophrenias.* New York: International Universities Press.

Boydell, J., Van Os, J., McKenzie, K., et al. (2001). Incidence of schizophrenia in ethnic minorities in London: Ecological study into interactions with environment. *British Medical Journal, 323,* 1336.

Carpenter, W. T., Heinrichs, D. W., & Wagman, A. M. (1988). Deficit and nondeficit forms of schizophrenia: The concept. *American Journal of Psychiatry, 145,* 578–583.

Chadwick, P., & Birchwood, M. (1994). Challenging the omnipotence of voices: A cognitive approach to auditory hallucinations. *British Journal of Psychiatry, 164,* 190–201.

Chadwick, P., Birchwood, M., & Trower, P. (1996). *Cognitive therapy of voices, delusions and paranoia.* Chichester, UK: Wiley.

Chadwick, P., Lees, S., & Birchwood, M. (2000). The revised Beliefs About Voices Questionnaire (BAVQ-R). *British Journal of Psychiatry, 177,* 229–232.

Chadwick, P., & Lowe, E. F. (1990). Measurement and modification of delusional beliefs. *Journal of Consulting and Clinical Psychology, 58,* 225–232.

Cox, D., & Cowling, P. (1989). *Are you normal?* London: Tower Press.

Crow, T. J. (1985). Molecular pathology of schizophrenia: More than one disease process? *British Medical Journal, 280,* 66–68.

Cunningham-Owens, D. G., Carroll, A., Fattah, S., et al. (2001). A randomized controlled trial of a brief interventional package for schizophrenic out-patients. *Acta Psychiatrica Scandinavica, 103,* 362–369.

David, A. S. (1990). Insight and psychosis. *British Journal of Psychiatry, 156,* 798–808.

Dickerson, F. B. (2000). Cognitive behavioral psychotherapy for schizophrenia: A review of recent empirical studies. *Schizophrenia Research, 43,* 71–90.

Drury, V., Birchwood, M., Cochrane, R., et al. (1996). Cognitive therapy and recovery from acute psychosis: A controlled trial: 1. Impact on psychotic symptoms. *British Journal of Psychiatry, 169,* 593–601.

Durham, R. C., Guthrie, M., Morton, R. V., et al. (2003). Tayside–Fife clinical trial of cognitive-behavioural therapy for medication-resistant psychotic symptoms: Results to 3-month follow-up. *British Journal of Psychiatry, 182,* 303–311.

Endicott, J., Spitzer, R. L., Fleiss, J. L., et al. (1976). The global assessment scale. A procedure for measuring overall severity of psychiatric disturbance. *Archives of General Psychiatry, 33,* 766–771.

Falloon, I. R. H., Boyd, J. L., McGill, C. W., et al. (1985). Family management in the prevention of morbidity of schizophrenia: Clinical outcome of a two-year longitudinal study. *Archives of General Psychiatry, 42,* 887–896.

Fowler, D., Garety, P., & Kuipers, L. (1995). *Cognitive therapy of psychoses.* Chichester, UK: Wiley.

Fowler, D., & Morley, S. (1989). The cognitive behavioural treatment of hallucinations and delusions: A preliminary study. *Behavioural Psychotherapy, 17,* 267–282.

Gath, D. H., & Mynors-Wallis, L. M. (1997). Problem-solving treatment in primary care. In D. M.

Clark & C. G. Fairburn (Eds.), *Science and practice of cognitive behaviour therapy*. Oxford: Oxford University Press.

Garety, P., Fowler, D., Kuipers, E., et al. (1997). London-East Anglia randomised controlled trial of cognitive-behavioural therapy for psychosis: II. Predictors of outcome. *British Journal of Psychiatry, 171*, 420–426.

Garety, P., & Freeman, D. (1999). Cognitive approaches to delusions: A critical review of theories and evidence. *British Journal of Clinical Psychology, 38*(2), 113–154.

Garety, P., & Hemsley, D. R. (1994). Delusions: Investigations into the psychology of delusional reasoning. *Maudsley Monograph*. Oxford: Oxford University Press.

Garety, P., Kuipers, E., Fowler, D., et al. (1994). Cognitive behavioural therapy for drug resistant psychosis. *British Journal of Medical Psychology, 67*(3), 259–271.

Garety, P., Kuipers, E., Fowler, D., et al. (2001). Cognitive model of the positive symptoms of psychosis. *Psychological Medicine, 31*(2), 189–195.

Geddes, J., Freemantle, N., Harrison, P., et al. (2000). Atypical antipsychotics in the treatment of schizophrenia: Systematic overview and metaregression analysis. *British Medical Journal, 321*(7273), 1371–6.

Geddes, J. R., & Lawrie, S. M. (1995). Obstetric complications and schizophrenia: A meta-analysis. *British Journal of Psychiatry, 167*, 786–793.

Gould, R. A., Mueser, K. T., et al. (2001). Cognitive therapy for psychosis in schizophrenia: An effect size analysis. *Schizophrenia Research, 48*, 335–342.

Groves, T. (1990). After the asylums: The local picture. *British Medical Journal, 300*, 1128–30.

Gumley, A., O'Grady, M., & McNay, L. (2003). Early intervention for relapse in schizophrenia: Results of a 12-month randomized controlled trial of cognitive behavoural therapy. *Psychological Medicine, 33*, 419–431.

Haddock, G., Bentall, R. P., & Slade, P. D. (1996). Psychological treatment of auditory hallucinations: Focusing or distraction? In G. Haddock & P. D. Slade (Eds.), *Cognitive Behavioural Interventions with Psychotic Disorders*. London: Routledge.

Haddock, G., McCarron, J., Tarrier, N., & Faragher, E. B. (1999). Scales to measure dimensions of hallucinations and delusions: The psychotic symptom rating scales (PSYRATS). *Psychological Medicine, 29*, 879–889.

Haddock, G., Sellwood, W., Tarrier, N., et al. (1994). Developments in cognitive behavioural therapy for persistent psychotic symptoms. *Behaviour Change, 11*(4), 200–212.

Hamilton, M. (1984). *Fish's schizophrenia* (3rd ed.). Bristol, UK: Wright.

Harrison, G., Hopper, K., Craig, T., et al. (2001). Recovery from psychotic illness: A 15 and 25 year international follow-up study. *British Journal of Psychiatry, 178*, 506–517.

Harrow, M., & Prosen, M. (1978). Intermingling and disordered logic as influences on schizophrenic "thought disorders." *Archives of General Psychiatry, 35*, 1213–1218.

Heins, T., Gray, A., & Tennant, M. (1990). Persisting hallucinations following childhood sexual abuse. *Australian and New Zealand Journal of Psychiatry, 24*, 561–565.

Hemsley, D. R., & Garety, P. A. (1986). The formation and maintenance of delusions: A Bayesian analysis. *British Journal of Psychiatry, 149*, 51–56.

Hirsch, S. R., & Jolley, A. G. (1989). The dysphoric syndrome in schizophrenia and its implications for relapse. *British Journal of Psychiatry, 155*(Suppl. 5), 46–50.

Hogarty, G. E., Anderson, C. M., Reiss, D. J., et al. (1991). Family psychoeducation, social skills training and maintenance chemotherapy in the after care treatment of schizophrenia: II. Two year effects of a controlled study on relapse and adjustment. *Archives of General Psychiatry, 48*, 340–347.

Hogarty, G. E., Kornblith, S. J., Greenwald, D., et al. (1997). Three year trials of personal therapy among schizophrenic patients living with or independent of family: I. Description of study and effects of relapse rates. *American Journal of Psychiatry, 154*(11), 1504–1513.

Hole, R. W., Rush, A. J., & Beck, A. T. (1979). A cognitive investigation of schizophrenic delusions. *Psychiatry, 42*, 312–319.

Jaspers, K. (1963). *General Psychopathology* (J. Hoenig & M. N. Hamilton, Trans.). Manchester: Manchester University Press.

Johns, L. C., & Van Os, J. (2001). The continuity of psychotic experiences in the general population. *Clinical Psychology Review, 21*, 1125–1141.

Jones, C., Cormac, I., Mota, J., & Campbell, C. (1999). *Cognitive Behaviour Therapy for Schizophrenia (Cochrane Review), Issue 4.* Oxford: Update Software.

Kane, J., Honigfeld, G., Singer, J., et al. (1988). Clozapine for the treatment-resistant schizophrenic. A double-blind comparison with chlorpromazine. *Archives of General Psychiatry, 45*, 789–96.

Kay, S., Fiszbein, A., & Opler, L. (1987). The Positive and Negative Syndrome Scale (PANSS) for schizophrenia. *Schizophrenia Bulletin, 13*, 261–275.

Keenan, B. (1992). *An Evil Cradling.* London: Arrow.

Kemp, R., Hayward, P., Applewhaite, G., Everitt, B., & David, A. (1996). Compliance therapy in psychotic peoples: A randomised controlled study. *British Medical* Journal, *312*, 345–349.

Kemp, R., Kirov, G., Everitt, B., et al. (1998). A randomised controlled trial of compliance therapy: 18-month follow-up. *British Journal of Psychiatry, 172*, 413–419.

Kingdon, D. G., & Turkington, D. (1991). The use of cognitive behavior therapy with a normalizing rationale in schizophrenia: Preliminary report. *Journal of Nervous and Mental Disease, 179*(4), 207–211.

Kingdon, D. G., & Turkington, D. (1994). *Cognitive behavior therapy of schizophrenia.* New York: Guilford Press.

Kingdon, D. G., & Turkington, D. (1998). Cognitive behavioural therapy of schizophrenia: Styles and methods. In T. Wykes, N. Tarrier, & S. F. Lewis (Eds.), *Outcome and innovation in psychological treatment of schizophrenia.* Chichester, UK: Wiley.

Kingdon, D. G., & Turkington, D. (2002). *A case study guide to cognitive therapy of psychosis.* Chichester, UK: Wiley.

Kingdon, D. G., Turkington, D., Collis, J., et al. (1989). Befriending schemes: Cost-effective community care. *Psychiatric Bulletin, 13*, 350–351.

Kingdon, D. G., Turkington, D., & John, C. (1994). Cognitive behaviour therapy of schizophrenia. *British Journal of Psychiatry, 164*, 581–587.

Krawiecka, M., Goldberg, G., & Vaughan, M. (1977). A standardized psychiatric assessment for rating chronic psychiatric patients. *Acta Psychiatrica Scandinavica, 55*, 299–308.

Kuipers, E., Fowler, D., Garety, P., et al. (1998). London-East Anglia randomised controlled trial of cognitive-behavioural therapy for psychosis: III. Follow-up and economic evaluation at 18 months. *British Journal of Psychiatry, 173*, 6168.

Kuipers, E., Garety, P., Fowler, D., et al. (1997). London-East Anglia randomised controlled trial of cognitive-behavioural therapy for psychosis: 1. Effects of the treatment phase. *British Journal of Psychiatry, 171*, 319–327.

Lecompte, D., & Pelc, I. (1996). A cognitive behavioral program to improve compliance with medication in peoples with schizophrenia. *International Journal of Mental Health, 25*, 51–56.

Leff, J. P. (1968). Perceptual phenomena and personality in sensory deprivation. *British Journal of Psychiatry, 114*, 1499–1508.

Leff, J., Kuipers, L., Berkowitz, R., & Sturgeon, D. (1985). A controlled trial of social intervention in the families of schizophrenic patients: Two year follow-up. *British Journal of Psychiatry, 146*, 594–600.

Lewis, S. W., Tarrier, N., Haddock, G., et al. (2002). A randomised controlled trial of cognitive-behaviour therapy in early schizophrenia: Acute phase outcomes in the SoCRATES trial. *British Journal of Psychiatry, 181*(43), s91–97.

Liddle, P. F., & Barnes, T. R. (1990). Syndromes of chronic schizophrenia. *British Journal of Psychiatry, 157*, 558–561.

McCreadie, R. G., & Robinson, A. D. (1987). The Nithsdale Schizophrenia Survey VI, Relatives' Expressed Emotion: Prevalence, Patterns, and Clinical Assessment. *British Journal of Psychiatry, 150*, 640–644.

McGorry, P., Edwards, S., Milhalopolous, M., et al. (1996). EPPIC: An evolving system of early detection and optimal management. *Schizophrenia Bulletin, 22*, 305–326.

McGorry, P. D., Yung, A. R., Phillips, L. J., et al. (2002). Randomized controlled trial of interventions designed to reduce the risk of progression to first-episode psychosis in a clinical sample with subthreshold symptoms. *Archives of General Psychiatry, 59*, 921–928.

Meichenbaum, D. (1969). The effects of instructions and reinforcement on thinking and language behaviour of schizophrenics. *Behaviour Research and Therapy, 7*, 101–114.

Meichenbaum, D., & Cameron, R. (1973). Training schizophrenics to talk to themselves: A means of developing attentional controls. *Behaviour Therapy, 4*, 515–534.

Milton, R., Patwa, V. K., & Hafner, R. J. (1978). Confrontation vs. belief modification in persistently deluded patients. *British Journal of Psychology, 4*, 235–242.

Morrison, A. P. (1998). A cognitive analysis of the maintenance of auditory hallucinations: Are voices to schizophrenia what bodily sensations are to panic? *Behavioural and Cognitive Psychotherapy, 26*, 289–302.

Morrison, A. P. (2001). The interpretation of intrusions in psychosis: An integrative cognitive approach to hallucinations and delusions. *Behavioural and Cognitive Psychotherapy, 29*, 257–276..

Morrison, A. P., Bentall, R. P., French, P., et al. (2002). Randomised controlled trial of early detection and cognitive therapy for preventing transition to psychosis in high-risk individuals: Study design and interim analysis of transition rate and psychological risk factors. *British Journal of Psychiatry, 43*, s78–84.

National Institute for Clinical Excellence. (2002). Clinical Guideline: 1. Schizophrenia. (*www.nice.org.uk*—accessed November 14, 2003).

Oswald, I. (1974). *Sleep* (3rd ed.). Harmondsworth, UK: Penguin.

Overall, J. E., & Gorham, D. R. (1962). The brief psychiatric rating scale. *Psychological Reports, 10*, 799–812.

Pekkala, E., & Merinder, L. (2000). *Psycheducational interventions for schizophrenia and other severe mental illnesses*. Oxford: Update Software.

Persons, J. B. (1986). The advantages of studying psychological phenomena rather than psychiatric diagnoses. *American Psychologist, 41*, 1252–1260.

Pilling, P., Bebbington, P., Kuipers, E., et al. (2002). Psychological treatments in schizophrenia: I. Meta-analysis of family interventions and cognitive-behaviour therapy. *Psychological Medicine, 32*, 763–782.

Pinto, A., La Pia, S., Mennella, R., et al. (1999). Cognitive-behavioral therapy for clozapine clients with treatment-refractory schizophrenia. *Psychiatric Services, 50*, 901–904.

Rachman, S., & de Silva, P. (1978). Abnormal and normal obsessions. *Behaviour Research and Therapy, 16*(4), 233–248.

Rathod, S., Kingdon, D., & Turkington, D. (2003). *Insight and schizophrenia*. Presentation at Psychological Interventions in Schizophrenia Conference, Oxford.

Rector, N. A., & Beck, A. T. (2001). Cognitive behavioral therapy for schizophrenia: an empirical review. *Journal of Nervous and Mental Disease, 189*, 278–287.

Rector, N. A., Seeman, M. V., & Segal, Z. V. (2003). Cognitive therapy of schizophrenia: A preliminary randomized controlled trial. *Schizophrenia Research, 63*, 1–11.

Roberts, G. A. (1991). Delusional systems and meaning in life—a preferred reality? *British Journal of Psychiatry, 14*, 20–29.

Robson, P. (1989). Development of a new self-report questionnaire to measure self-esteem. *Psychological Medicine, 19,* 513–518.

Romme, M., & Escher, A. (1989). Hearing voices. *Schizophenia Bulletin, 15,* 209–216.

Ross, C. A., Anderson, G., & Clark, P. (1994). Childhood abuse and positive symptoms of schizophrenia. *Hospital and Community Psychiatry, 45,* 489–491.

Salokangas, R., Rakkolainen, V., Stengard, E., et al. (1991). *Usien Skitsofreniapotilaiden Hoito ja Ennuste: 5 Vuoden Seuranta.* Helsinki: Psykiatrian Tutkimussaatio.

Scott, J., Byers, S., & Turkington, D. (1992). The chronic patient. In J. Wright (Ed.), *Cognitive therapy with inpatients.* New York: Guilford Press.

Sensky, T., Turkington, D., Kingdon, D., et al. (2000). A randomised controlled trial of cognitive-behavioural therapy for persistent symptoms in schizophrenia resistant to medication. *Archives of General Psychiatry, 57,* 165–172.

Strauss, J. S. (1969). Hallucinations and delusions as points on continua function. *Archives of General Psychiatry, 21,* 581–586.

Strauss, J. S. (1989). Mediating processes in schiziphrenia. *British Journal of Psychiatry, 155*(5), S22–S28.

Tarrier, N., Barrowclough, C., Vaughn, C., et al. (1989). Community management of schizophrenia. A two-year follow-up of a behavioural intervention with families. *British Journal of Psychiatry, 154,* 625–628.

Tarrier, N., Beckett, R., Harwood, S., et al. (1993). A trial of two cognitive behavioural methods of treating drug resistant residual symptoms in schizophrenic peoples: I. Outcome. *British Journal of Psychiatry, 162,* 524–532.

Tarrier, N., Harwood, S., Yussof, L., et al. (1990). Coping strategy enhancement (C.S.E.): A method of treating residual schizophrenic symptoms. *Behavioural Psychotherapy, 18,* 643–662.

Tarrier, N., Kinney, C., McCarthy, E., et al. (2001). Are some types of psychotic symptoms more responsive to cognitive behaviour therapy? *Behavioural and Cognitive Psychotherapy, 29,* 45–55.

Tarrier, N., Lewis, S. W., Haddock, G., et al. (2004). Cognitive-behavioural therapy in first-episode and early schizophrenia: 18-month follow-up of a randomised controlled trial. *British Journal of Psychiatry, 184,* 231–239.

Tarrier, N., Wittowski, A., Kinney, C., et al. (1999). Durability of the effects of cognitive-behavioural therapy in the treatment of chronic schizophrenia: 12 month follow up. *British Journal of Psychiatry, 174,* 500–504.

Tarrier, N., Yusupoff, L, Kinney, C., et al. (1998). Randomised controlled trial of intensive cognitive behaviour therapy for patients with chronic schizophrenia. *British Medical Journal, 317,* 303–307.

Turkington, D., John, C. H., Siddle, R., et al. (1996). Cognitive therapy in the treatment of drug resistant delusional disorder. *Clinical Psychology and Psychotherapy, 3,* 118–128.

Turkington, D., & Kingdon, D. G. (1991). Ordering thoughts in thought disorder. *British Journal Psychiatry, 159,* 160–161.

Turkington, D, & Kingdon, D. G. (1996). The use of a normalising rationale in schizophrenia. In G. Haddock & P. D. Slade (Eds.), *Cognitive-Behavioural Interventions with Psychotic Disorders.* London: Routledge.

Turkington, D., Kingdon, D. G., Turner, T., et al. (2002). The Insight Programme: Effectiveness of a brief cognitive-behavioural intervention in the treatment of schizophrenia. *British Journal of Psychiatry, 180,* 523–7.

Turkington, D., & Siddle, R. (1998). Cognitive therapy for the treatment of delusions. *Advances in Psychiatric Treatment, 4,* 235–242.

Vaughn, C., & Leff, J. (1976). The influence of family and social factors on the course of psychiatric illness. A comparison of schizophrenia and depressed neurotic patients. *British Journal of Psychiatry, 129,* 125–137.

Verdoux, H., Geddes, J. R., Takei, N., et al. (1997). Obstetric complications and age at onset in schizophrenia: An international collaborative meta-analysis of individual patient data. *American Journal of Psychiatry, 154*(9), 1220–1227.

Walsh, E., Moran, P., Scott, K., et al. (2003). Prevalence of violent victimisation in severe mental illness. *British Journal of Psychiatry, 183*, 233–238.

Wing, J. K., Beevor, A. S., Curtis, R. H., et al. (1998). A Health of the Nation Outcome Scale (HoNOS): Research and development. *British Journal of Psychiatry, 172*, 11–18.

Wing, J. K., Curtis, R. H., & Beevor, A. S. (1996). *HoNOS: Health of the Nation Outcome Scales: Report on research and development, July 1993–December 1995.* London: Royal College of Psychiatrists.

World Health Organization. (1992). *International classification of diseases* (10th ed.). Geneva: Author.

Young, J., & Beck, A. T. (1980). *Cognitive Therapy Scale.* Unpublished manuscript.

Further Readings

Barrowclough, C., & Tarrier, N. (1992). *Families of schizophrenic persons: Cognitive behavioral intervention.* London: Chapman & Hall.

Beck, A. T. (1976). *Cognitive therapy of the emotional disorders.* New York: International Universities Press.

Bentall, R. P. (2003). *Madness explained.* London: Allen Lane, Penguin Press.

Birchwood M., Jackson C., Fowler, D. (2000). *Early Intervention in psychosis: A guide to concepts, evidence and Interventions.* Chichester: Wiley.

Clarke, I. (2001). *Psychosis and spirituality: Exploring the new frontier.* London: Whurr.

French, P., & Morrison, A. P. (2004). *Early detection and cognitive therapy for people at high risk of developing psychosis.* Chichester, UK: Wiley.

Graham, H. L., Mueser, K., Birchwood, M. J., et al. (2002). *Substance Misuse in Psychosis—Approaches to Treatment and Service Delivery.* Chichester, UK: Wiley.

Morrison, A. P. (2002). *A casebook of cognitive therapy for psychosis.* Hove, UK: Routledge.

Nelson, H. (1997). *Cognitive behavioral therapy with schizophrenia: A practice manual.* London: Stanley Thornes.

Tarrier, N., Wells, A., & Haddock, G. (1998). *Treating complex cases: The cognitive behavioral therapy approach.* Chichester, UK: Wiley.

Index

U

V

W